THE
Autoimmune
PLAGUE

THE
Autoimmune
PLAGUE

*How to
Regain Sovereignty
over Your Body and Life*

Dr. Colby Kash, D.C., M.S.

White River Press
Amherst, Massachusetts

First published 2022 by White River Press
Amherst, Massachusetts 01004 • whiteriverpress.com

Book and cover design by Lufkin Graphic Designs
Norwich, Vermont 05055 • www.LufkinGraphics.com

The contents of this book are for informational purposes only, and are not intended to diagnose or treat any medical condition, and should not replace professional medical advice. You should seek the advice of a physician or other health care professional for any questions you may have regarding a medical condition. I caution you not to disregard professional medical advice, or in any way delay seeking medical attention, based on the contents of this book.

ISBN: 978-1-935052-89-0 (paperback)
       978-1-935052-94-4 (ebook)

Library of Congress Cataloging-in-Publication Data

Names: Kash, Colby, 1995- author.
Title: The autoimmune plague : regain sovereignty over your body and life /
   Dr. Colby Kash, D.C., M.S.
Description: Amherst, Massachusetts : White River Press, [2022] | Includes
   bibliographical references and index. | Summary: "A science-based
   blueprint of the author's journey back to health from autoimmune
   disease: not one, but three classified autoimmune diseases. It is his
   mission to empower and educate as many people as possible to take
   control of their health. He presents the proprietary to decreasing the
   common autoimmune triggers, increasing the body's resilience, and
   preventing reoccurrence. The Autoimmune Plague provides evidence-based
   changes to diet, lifestyle, and gives awareness to alternative
   therapies/technologies that many doctors are unlikely to be trained in
   or share with patients"-- Provided by publisher.
Identifiers: LCCN 2022017165 | ISBN 9781935052890 (trade paperback)
Subjects: LCSH: Kash, Colby, 1995---Health. | Autoimmune
   diseases--Alternative treatment. | Autoimmune
   diseases--Patients--Biography. | Self-care, Health.
Classification: LCC RC600 .K36 2022 | DDC 616.97/8--dc23/eng/20220713
LC record available at https://lccn.loc.gov/2022017165

Acknowledgements

To my mother for unconditional love and support through every stage of my life.

To my father for expanding my mind about what can be possible and leading by example.

To Jared, Shantal, and Zena for always being in my corner.

To past mentors and coaches for teaching me important life lessons.

To those suffering with autoimmune conditions, this book is for you.

Contents

My Story and The History of Autoimmune Disease

"Illnesses do not come upon us out of the blue. They are developed from small daily sins against nature. When enough sins have accumulated, illnesses will suddenly appear."

—Hippocrates

ONE MORNING I AWOKE IN A COLD SWEAT, as a sharp dagger of pain reverberated through my body. I was alarmed to find my hands swollen to the size of baseballs; I had no recollection of any trauma. The next day the swelling progressed to my elbows and fingers. Then, the restricting pain had caught up to my hips, knees, and feet. I was officially rendered useless and called out of work sick. I lay bedridden in a prison that had been beautifully designed by my immune system. My body was at war, at war with itself. In just a few days, how did I transform into moving like a 90-year-old grandma with a tennis-ball-bottomed walker? The answer was interwoven not only in my lifestyle, but in the same way YOU—and all of us—live in twenty-first-century Western civilization.

As far back as I can remember, I always had a wonky digestive system. Around twelve years of age, I was riddled with painful stomachaches, gas, bloating, and frequent staycations to the stall. I had seen a multitude of conventional doctors of varying specialties. However, I had never been given a treatment protocol or an explanation of what might be causing the symptoms or suggestions on what to do about it. Instead, I was slapped with the label IBS (Irritable Bowel Syndrome), a diagnosis of exclusion and synonymous with they don't know what's going on. I even remember a doctor suggesting that I should "attempt a bowel movement after dinner," as if that was sound medical advice. Another doctor dispassionately explained that it was normal to live with a "dysfunctional" stomach. Unfortunately, this happens too often when patients see their doctor for symptoms that don't show up on a blood test, and the doctor simply dismisses it as normal.

As the years went on, my symptoms progressed into bloody stools and gut-wrenching pain. Inflammation in the gut had spread to my skin in the form of acne and psoriasis, and it systematically evolved into bouts of brain fog, achy joints, and low mood. At the age of 24, "IBS" had progressed to the diagnosis of Crohn's disease, whereby my immune system was attacking my gut lining and microbiota. I was put on a relatively safe drug called Mesalamine. However, my body had different plans and expressed an adverse reaction to the drug. It taught me a whole new meaning of the word nausea and ultimately lead to the next progression of the disease, psoriatic arthritis, as colorfully described with the dominoing of inflammation from my fingers to my toes. Yet another heap of stress piled into the stress bank that had tipped my body into bathing my joints with inflammation. My insides were now fighting a multi-front war with its newest flank ambushing the synovium of my joints.

While in Chiropractic School, I began to study Nutrition and Functional Medicine, and I learned about the root cause of disease. In fact, I became obsessed, reading and listening to anything I could get my hands and ears on. I learned early on that I needed to take complete personal responsibility and extreme ownership of my autoimmune disease. I decided if I was going to be a doctor worth my salt, I had no choice but to relieve myself from the unknown, "incurable disease." While on that health journey, I gave birth to an autoimmune protocol that won the high ground at every known angle that this disease penetrates. Thankfully, I now thrive without the symptoms that once held me back.

How could autoimmune disease like this happen to such a young person who ate healthily and exercised regularly? Whether or not I knew what I was doing at the time, I had given myself Crohn's disease. I was consuming foods chalked with glyphosates, antibiotics, GMOS, BPA, among thousands of other chemicals. As a high-charging scholar/athlete, through academics, athletics, and extracurriculars at the highest levels, I was absorbing the stressors of life without finding time to wind down the mind through meditation. I was dousing myself with toxic shampoos and conditioners, binge drinking at college parties, and consuming high levels of sugar, plant defense toxins, and rancid vegetable oils.

What I didn't know at the time is that the body can't tell the difference between different stressors. It stockpiles them all into what I like to conceptualize as a stress bank. One can continue to deposit stress in its many different forms until it hits a predetermined amount and a gene for disease is turned on. As I continued to add more stressors, more cells began to express the diseased gene's phenotype. This is clinically referred to as allostatic load. Allostatic load is the price that the body pays for being forced to adapt to stressful situations. The body's ultimate goal is to always return to homeostasis or your body's baseline. Under normal circumstances the body has its most efficient baseline heart rate, body temperature, and blood pressure, along with thousands of other metrics, some of which work in cycles. However, chronic exposures to elevated levels of endocrine, neural, or other chemical signals can prevent the return to homeostasis. These signals are part of the language that the body uses to express stress to its cells.

In times of heavy stress, the body will always protect its most important functions. For example, during cold exposure, it will keep your internal organs heated at the expense of your little piggies. Or during an infection, the body will turn on its internal thermostat to kill the potentially life-threatening pathogen at the risk of denaturing our own proteins! From a chemical messenger perspective, when both histamine and adrenaline are concomitantly released, adrenaline's signal overrides that of histamine in cells. This is because histamine is simply a local response, whereas adrenaline's systemic effect can be a result of something much more life-threatening. The adrenal surge from a lion chasing after you is more important than increasing swelling at the site of a bug bite or infection. Very quickly you can see how chronic stress can alter the body's priorities.

Autoimmune disease is caused by compounding stressors and immune dysregulation. A smorgasbord of psychological, emotional, physical, and environmental stresses all play into the synergistic chronic drag on the body. Evolutionally, the human body was designed to deal with acute bouts of fight-or-flight situations in nature and then wobble back into homeostasis. We are designed to have a certain level of stress resilience. Acute stressors provide tremendous benefit to the body, such as exercise, sauna, cold thermogenesis, plant toxins, ozone, etc. In modern times, many of us live in overwhelming comfort and avoid building our bodies up to be able to grapple with stress. Immune dysregulation begins when the bad microorganisms within us begin to outgrow the good ones. These microorganisms speak to our cells through chemical messages. Most importantly, these messages can code for the downregulation or upregulation of inflammation. Other chemical messages can even act as food substrates for our cells. Another cause of immune dysregulation includes the deficiency of certain micronutrients that build up our defenses and manufacture immune-fighting cells. Thus, we must optimize our microecosystems to create a homeostatic and harmonious environment.

Learning about how our world interacts with our immune system empowered me to speak to my own immune system in ways that it can understand. In later chapters, I have outlined potential immune triggers and how to identify the stressors and effectively eliminate them from your stress bank. Once healed, you will learn how to select which environmental factors to reintroduce back into your life. Sometimes just eliminating a few triggers, as in my case, is not enough. While we eliminate triggers, we must simultaneously finance our body's antioxidant and detoxification systems to speed up recovery and help win back the tug-of-war with your immune system. I also delve into the supplements, modalities, and lifestyle practices that will help you facilitate this process.

You are the CEO of your health; nobody can heal you but you! The first step is accepting that your lifestyle and past decisions, even ones you once thought were safe, contributed to your autoimmune disease. In all but extremely rare cases, we are not born with autoimmune disease. Rather, it is an epigenetic manifestation of interactions in our environment. With the right inspiration and knowledge, you can manufacture an epigenetic milieu full of conscious lifestyle decisions that will get your health back in order.

Although this might seem like an emotional journey, try not to dwell on the question "why me?" Rather, feel blessed that you live in an information era where the right knowledge and tools are right in front of you. This book is a guide to your journey back to optimal health. And though there will be up and downs, make this journey your new purpose in life. It is going to require your full commitment and attention. However, through this process you will grow as an individual to new heights, both physically and spiritually, that you could not have achieved without a unique adversity. As the famous holocaust survivor and psychiatrist, Viktor Frankel, states in *Man's Search for Meaning*, "If there is meaning in life at all, then there must be meaning in suffering."

As you may imagine, we are not alone. There are between 23.5–50 million Americans suffering from the debilitating symptoms of autoimmune disease: up to one out of seven people. In fact, it is estimated that there are more than 100 autoimmune diseases.[1] The most well-known autoimmune diseases are Hashimoto's disease, Irritable Bowel Syndrome, Multiple Sclerosis, Psoriasis, Rheumatoid Arthritis, Sjogren's Syndrome, Type 1 Diabetes, and Celiac Disease. Patients with these autoimmunity diseases suffer debilitating symptoms of neurologic degeneration, vascular compromise, metabolic insufficiency, gut pathology, skin derangement, chronic inflammation, organ/tissue destruction, and loss of physical mobility as well as an increased likelihood of death. Autoimmune disease has transformed into a modern calamity, and its plague shadows the lives of hundreds of millions of people globally.

The United States spends 18 percent of its GDP on health care, and that number is continuing to creep up.[2] As much as 90 percent of the healthcare budget is expended on chronic health conditions.[3] In 2003, treatment cost and lost productivity amounted to $1.3 trillion.[4] Treatment of autoimmune conditions cost around $100 billion annually, which is likely a vast underestimation because autoimmune disorders are often conflated under other disease categories. The top seven autoimmune diseases alone account for $50–70 billion a year.[5] Without major reform, the cost of autoimmune disease and chronic illness will eventually cause our healthcare system to collapse.

Improvements in preventative care could completely offset this downward spiral; modest estimates suggest that preventative care could save hundreds of billions of dollars annually.[6] Just imagine what other social programs that money could be allocated toward, to benefit our great nation. Trends for autoimmunity are continuing to rise. Type 1 Diabetes has more than doubled in the last 30 years, and Celiac disease has tripled in the last decade alone.

In addition, 75 percent of people with autoimmune disease are women. The National Institute of Health's Office of Research on Women's Health has declared autoimmune disease a major women's health issue because it is one of the top 10 leading causes of death in women aged under 65, and is the 4th largest cause of disability for women.[7] One theory as to why women are more likely to suffer from autoimmune disease is that they have much higher levels of estrogen, which may influence immune signaling. Animal studies support this theory; they demonstrate that castrated males see elevated levels of autoimmunity, as do mice given inflated levels of estrogen. Testosterone given to Lupus-prone mice suppressed the effect of the disease.[8] It is possible that environmental estrogens in our foods, packaging, and cosmetic products may also be contributing. There are likely more pieces to the puzzle than just estrogen causing the differential between sex rates of autoimmunity.

The chronic nature of autoimmune disease contributes to extended absence from employment. Patients are slapped with expensive medical bills that, because of lost wages, they struggle to pay for. This illuminates the huge psychological/physical cost to a patient and society.

A survey published in the *Journal of Rheumatology* noted an average earnings' decrease in Rheumatoid Arthritis patients from $18,409–$13,900 per year. At the same time, the number of jobs that Rheumatoid Arthritis patients could perform dropped from 11.5 million to 2.6 million. Furthermore, within 10 years of disease onset, 50 percent of Rheumatoid Arthritis patients become unable to work at all.[9] This is the most common type of autoimmune disease in the United States. The human blow is not just debilitating on an individual level but is also a huge burden on the economy and affects the ability of the United States both to be competitive in global markets and to produce healthy candidates for our armed services.

The oldest cohort of individuals, people aged 85 or older, are the fastest-growing segment of the U.S. population. Currently numbering 4 million people, this segment of the population could surpass 19 million by 2050. In 1950, there were an estimated 3,000 American centenarians, whereas by 2050 there could be

1 million![10] The major 21st-century challenge is how to shift toward additional years of vibrant health and productivity versus the current trend of increasing disabilities, comorbidities, and decreased quality of life. Do we just want to live, or do we want to thrive?

One of the current trends has one in two women, and one in four men over age 50, breaking a bone due to osteoporosis.[11] Having an autoimmune disease increases the risk of osteoporosis, and there seems to be a role of autoantibodies in inflammatory osteoporosis.[12] As risk of osteoporosis rises so does Alzheimer's disease (AD), cardiovascular disease, cancer, and diabetes.[13, 14] Autoimmune disease can cause a cascading debilitating condition into other diseases. Many older Americans suffer from multiple health problems; these comorbidities tend to complicate treatments and severely decrease quality of life. When an individual has one autoimmune disease, their risk of another greatly increases. The inability to eliminate chronic low-grade inflammation associated with autoimmune disease will eventually allow for the overload of oxidative stress to be expressed as a new disease in the body.

From an evolutionary perspective, these diseases are not protective and therefore are most likely not naturally supposed to occur at the increasing rates we currently see. It is true that hunter-gathers died on average when they were 30 years old. However, they were exposed to the elements, had no emergency medical care, and had high rates of trauma, violence, warfare, and an infant and early childhood mortality that was 30 times higher than it is today. Contemporary hunter-gatherers who make it to age 45 can expect to live another 20 years and possibly into their 70s and beyond but without any of the chronic inflammatory diseases we experience: autoimmunity, allergies, asthma, heart disease, or diabetes.[15] This illuminates the modern variables in our lifestyle not seen in hunter-gatherers, which may be contributing to disease.

Over and over again, we've been told that autoimmune disease is largely determined by our genetics and that the root cause is unknown. This statement is misleading, leaving patients disempowered and full of self-doubt—a recipe for a hopeless downward physical and mental spiral that won't be eliminated by washing down a cocktail of immune suppressants. We all deserve better healthcare than this. The mainstream narrative is **WRONG**. Identical twin studies show that even with the same DNA and upbringing, autoimmunity can manifest in one twin and not the other![16] DNA may predispose us, but it does not write the prescription for illness. When humans decrease oxidative stress, symptoms of autoimmune disease begin to dissipate.[17] When the microbiome and vitamin deficiencies are normalized, the immune system returns to homeostasis and optimizes performance. Chronic disease is not created by our genetics but instead is largely environmental and behavioral. Our genes do play a role in determining which diseases we are predisposed to developing. However, the choices we make regarding diet, physical activity, sleep, stress management, and other lifestyle factors are far more important determinants of our health. Genes exist in a democracy with environmental signals.

There are 23,000 genes that make up the human genome with only about 0.1 percent gene variation between humans. These are the differences found in skin, hair, and eye color. I remember when I was in the cadaver lab in Chiropractic School and I was able to see that humans had more diversity internally than externally: whether it was an extra lobe of the lung, an absence of a particular muscle, or even an additional bone. However, through my research, I learned that most diversity that exists between humans lies somewhere we cannot see, in the immune system. Our immune cells have unique receptor shapes that explain our different responses to the same infection.

The same genes that cause autoimmune disease in Western civilization were protective in our ancient world. They are the genotype for a more aggressive immune response to infections and foreign bodies. In the presence of heavy stress and the absence of exposure to diverse bacteria and parasites, the body can mount a self-inflicted attack. One example is the HLA-B27 gene that predisposes Ankylosing Spondylitis, an autoimmune disease that causes a progressive fusion of spinal joints, but also slows the progress of HIV and Hepatitis C.[18] Another instance is those with a more resistant version of the STAT6 gene who have higher risk of allergies and asthma in Great Britain but lower parasite loads in China.[19] In Ghanaians, genes that increase inflammatory pathways also increase lifespan when living in an environment exposed to high amounts of microbes. However, simply take away river or well water and the pro-inflammatory gene variants decreased lifespan.[20] And then there is a filaggrin gene variant, which makes skin more porous. The theory is this gene allows for better communication with skin microbiota, giving more time to mount a counterattack. In today's environmental context, this gene correlates to skin inflammatory disorders.[21] It is important to remember that these specific genes work in cohesion with many other genes.

The conventional medical system seeks to treat chronic conditions such as autoimmunity by suppressing symptoms through drug usage. These drugs may or may not actually alleviate symptoms; they may or may not slow the progression of the disease. They may even make it worse and certainly won't reverse the disease.

The latest medical discoveries take an average of 17 years to reach clinical practice.[22] In conventional medicine, the doctor you see is likely a specialist in a specific organ. Since autoimmune diseases often affect multiple organs and systems in the body, teams of physicians including a Rheumatologist, Ophthalmologist, Neurologist, and Gastroenterologist often are needed to treat each individual symptom separately. If you want to address skin issues, the Dermatologist will seek to treat the inflammation in the skin; for thyroid problems you will see an Endocrinologist (who won't look past the glands); for your gut, a Gastroenterologist; and a Rheumatologist for your joints.

In certain circumstances, specialists only treat a specific part of an organ. This segmental approach misses the smoking gun commonality among them all. Functional Medicine is a comprehensive framework of medicine that incorporates all the organ systems intertwined into an interdependent biological ecosystem. It functions to treat the root cause of disease rather than to simply mask the symptoms or retard progression. Chronic low-grade inflammation is your body's systematic expression to stress, and suppressing the expression of a single organ is likely to simply pass the buck.

Modern medicine has made amazing strides in emergency medicine; however, it's been a huge failure when treating autoimmune and other chronic illnesses. The world's brightest minds have made incredible discoveries within immunology, but the emphasis has been misplaced. Drugs have their role but should not be the first and only line of defense. We must first support the most efficient drug producing pharmacy in the world, our bodies. Many physicians want to treat patients the right way but are held hostage to the reimbursements allowed by insurance companies. Evidence-based medicine does not give in to the pressures of Big Pharma and insurance companies, but rather uses all the tools in the right amounts at the right time.

I do want to clearly state that I am a proponent of Western medicine, and I believe that medications can be an important part of a holistic approach, especially for quelling initial inflammation. Our bodies and our immune systems did not evolve in an evolutionary-consistent environment and therefore may require modern pharmaceuticals (used at individualized dosages when appropriate) in conjunction to the tools provided in this book.

I also believe that there is a root cause of your autoimmune disease. I learned this the hard way because I had not one but three! Through personal experience, I was exposed to the true causes of autoimmune issues, and effectively eliminated them from my life with a holistic approach. I am dedicated to sharing this protocol in order to help as many people as possible become a healthier version of themselves. In this book, I will break down the immune system, the root cause of immune system dysfunction/autoimmune disease, the elimination of the common triggers, and how to accelerate the healing process and prevent the reoccurrence. I will refer to the entirety of the methodology as the Kash Code. Other autoimmune books promote how their protocol can help heal you in 30 days and this may be the case, but only in select individuals. While those books might talk about eliminating the low-hanging fruit such as dairy, gluten, or maybe even some plant toxins, for many people this won't even scratch the surface of recovery, as in my case, when they left me searching for more. This book is ideal for individuals that are self-driven to take control of their health but need the guidance and information to cross the finish line. It provides the radical diet modifications, radical lifestyle changes, and radical biohacks needed to make biochemical changes in the body. At the same time, the Kash Code does not shame patients for the use of pharmaceuticals when used appropriately in the holistic approach. My mission is to help you become the best version of yourself through the reversal of autoimmune disease: to eliminate the pain perturbing YOUR full potential and to help you regain sovereignty over YOUR body.

NOTES

1   *Rare autoimmune diseases: Individually rare, collectively common • aarda.* AARDA. (2019, Sept. 30). https://www.aarda.org/rare-autoimmune-diseases-individually-rare-collectively-common.

2   Elflein, J. (2020, June 8). *U.S. health spending as share of gdp 1960–2020.* Statista. https://www.statista.com/statistics/184968/us-health-expenditure-as-percent-of-gdp-since-1960.

3   Centers for Disease Control and Prevention. (2021, June 23). *Health and economic costs of chronic diseases.* Centers for Disease Control and Prevention. https://www.cdc.gov/chronicdisease/about/costs/index.htm.

4   *The costs of chronic disease in the U.S.: Milken Institute.* Chronic Disease Costs in the U.S. | Milken Institute Report. (n.d.). https://milkeninstitute.org/report/costs-chronic-disease-us.

5   Centers for Disease Control and Prevention. (2021, June 23). https://www.cdc.gov/chronicdisease/about/costs/index.htm.

6   *The costs of chronic disease in the U.S.: Milken Institute.* https://milkeninstitute.org/report/costs-chronic-disease-us.

7   Somnath Pal, B. S. P. (2016, June 16). *Trends in selected autoimmune diseases.* U.S. Pharmacist – The Leading Journal in Pharmacy. https://www.uspharmacist.com/article/trends-in-selected-autoimmune-diseases.

8   Desai, M. K. and Brinton, R. D. (2019, April 29). *Autoimmune disease in women: Endocrine transition and risk across the lifespan.* Frontiers in endocrinology. https://www.ncbi.nlm.nih.gov/pmc/articles/PMC6501433.

9   AARDA. (2011). *The Cost Burden of Autoimmune Disease: The Latest Front on the War Non-Healthcare Spending.* http://www.diabetesed.net/page/_files/autoimmune-diseases.pdf.   http://www.diabetesed.net/page/_files/autoimmune-diseases.pdf.

10   Bush, Elaine M., M. S. U. E. (2021, March 9). *As our population ages, unique challenges and needs continue to emerge.* MSU Extension. https://www.canr.msu.edu/news/as_our_population_ages_unique_challenges_and_needs_continue_to_emerge.

11   National Osteoporosis Foundation. *Osteoporosis Facts.* https://cdn.nof.org/wp-content/uploads/2015/12/Osteoporosis-Fast-Facts.pdf.

12   Iseme, R. A.; Mcevoy, M.; Kelly, B.; Agnew, L.; Walker, F. R.; Attia, J. (2017, Oct. 16). *Is osteoporosis an autoimmune mediated disorder?* Bone reports. https://www.ncbi.nlm.nih.gov/pmc/articles/PMC5671387.

13   Warburton, D. E. R.; Nicol, C. W.; Gatto, S. N.; Bredin, S. S. D. (2007). *Cardiovascular disease and osteoporosis: Balancing risk management.* Vascular health and risk management. https://www.ncbi.nlm.nih.gov/pmc/articles/PMC2291312.

14   Chen, Yu-Hung and Raymond Y Lo. "Alzheimer's Disease and Osteoporosis." *Ci Ji Yi Xue Za Zhi = Tzu-Chi Medical Journal*, Medknow Publications & Media Pvt. Ltd., 2017, www.ncbi.nlm.nih.gov/pmc/articles/PMC5615992.

15   Pontzer, H., et al. "Hunter-Gatherers as Models in Public Health." *Wiley Online Library*, John Wiley & Sons, Ltd, 3 Dec. 2018, onlinelibrary.wiley.com/doi/full/10.1111/obr.12785.

16   Rappaport, Stephen M. "Genetic Factors Are Not the Major Causes of Chronic Diseases." *PloS One*, Public Library of Science, 22 April 2016, www.ncbi.nlm.nih.gov/pmc/articles/PMC4841510.

17   *The influence of reactive oxygen species in the immune system and pathogenesis of multiple sclerosis.* Read by QxMD. Retrieved from https://read.qxmd.com/read/32789026/the-influence-of-reactive-oxygen-species-in-the-immune-system-and-pathogenesis-of-multiple-sclerosis?sid=48b73760-4d08-4736-8376-2c5a9b2c4d96%29.

18   Neumann-Haefelin, C.; Oniangue-Ndza, C.; Kuntzen, T.; Schmidt, J.; Nitschke, K.; Sidney, J.; Caillet-Saguy, C.; Binder, M.; Kersting, N.; Kemper, M. W.; Power, K. A.; Ingber, S.; Reyor, L. L.; Hills-Evans, K.; Kim, A. Y.; Lauer, G. M.; Lohmann, V.; Sette, A.; Henn, M. R.; Allen, T. M. (2011, October). *Human leukocyte antigen B27 selects for rare escape mutations that significantly impair hepatitis C virus replication and require compensatory mutations.* Hepatology (Baltimore, Md.). Retrieved Oct. 11, 2021, from https://www.ncbi.nlm.nih.gov/pmc/articles/PMC3201753.

19   Moller, M.; Gravenor, M. B.; Roberts, S. E.; Sun, D.; Gao. P.; Hopkin, J. M. (n.d.). *Genetic haplotypes of th-2 immune signalling link allergy*

to enhanced protection to parasitic worms. Human molecular genetics. Retrieved Oct. 11, 2021, from https://pubmed.ncbi.nlm.nih.gov/17519224.

20   Kuningas, Maris, et al. *Among Ghanaians living in a highly infectious . . .* "Selection for Genetic Variation Inducing Pro-inflammatory Responses Under Adverse Environmental Conditions in a Ghanaian Population," *PLoS ONE* 4, no. 11 (2009).

21   de Benedetto, A., et al. *Experiments firmly established*: "Tight Junction Defects in Patients with Atopic Dermatitis." *Journal of Allergy and Clinical Immunology,* 127, no. 3 (2011).

22   Morris, Z. S.; Wooding, S.; Grant, J. (2011, Dec.) *The answer is 17 years, what is the question: Understanding time lags in translational research.* Journal of the Royal Society of Medicine. Retrieved from https://www.ncbi.nlm.nih.gov/pmc/articles/PMC3241518.

CHAPTER 1

The Immune System

Before we can learn how to heal the immune system, it is of utmost importance to understand the innerworkings of the immune system, how all the different cells and chemical messengers work together, and then finally, where dysfunction begins to stem from. Throughout the book, I frequently refer back to this chapter in order to explain how a lifestyle or dietary change can modulate the immune system. If you have no interest in understanding the immune system on a micro level, you can skip this chapter.

THE IMMUNE SYSTEM is spread across the entire human body and functions to identify self from non-self in order to rid it of harmful bacteria, viruses, parasites, and fungi. The immune system also performs maintenance on dead and dysfunctional cells.

There are two types of immunity: the innate and the adaptive immune systems.

We are all born with the innate immune system, which gives our bodies the ability to fight foreign invaders from day one. The innate immunity includes the external barriers of our body such as skin, mucous membranes, and the gut lining. It functions as the first detection of pathogens. The immediate response is nonspecific and lacks immunologic memory of the bad guys. Of the millions of species known on earth, well over 90 percent of them survive with just the innate immune system, which also makes up the majority of defenses in humans.[1]

The adaptive immune system protects us from the foreign invaders as we grow through our lifetime. The immune information is gained through exposure to disease and vaccination, which builds up an arsenal of antibodies for all types of pathogens. Our adaptive immunity can store memory, thus allowing it to mount a rapid and efficient attack during future exposures. It automatically turns on if the innate immune system cannot effectively eliminate the pathogen.

The first line of defense in the innate immune system is the epithelial surfaces, which exist as skin on our exterior and lines our internal hollow organs. The skin, a frequently shedding thick coat of dead cells, acts as a selective barrier to keep antigens out. Antigens can take form as bacteria, toxins, virus, foreign tissues, or abnormal body cells. The skin produces antimicrobial proteins, oils, and other immune cells. Our digestive system produces a highly acidic and enzymatic environment to kill microbes off. Other areas of exposure like the eyes produce enzymes in tears, or the vagina that has antibacterial excretion. There are antibodies in the mucus linings of your respiratory and digestive tracts as preventative steps to ward off microscopic predators.[2] Even the anatomical engineering is perfected for tower defense. The nose has bones designed to create turbulence to filter dust, molds, and toxins, while larger particles are transported out of the respiratory system via cilia.[3]

Urinary and reproductive tracts are specially designed to prevent infections with a coating of mucous as well as by having a heavy presence of innate immunity and sterility. Similar to the importance of averting contamination from entering the body is the significance of toxic waste being excreted from our bodies. After the initial barrier defense, the body's next gear kicks in when a pathogen sneaks by. This includes the induction of a fever to use high temperatures to kill microbes, the release of chemical signals, inflammation, and a boost in cellular metabolism. When the immune cells become overwhelmed by high levels of pathogens, they release pyrogen chemicals that stimulate the pituitary gland to raise the body's systematic temperature. Other inflammatory chemical signals have fancy names like fatty acid prostaglandins, kininogen, plasma proteins, histamine, and cytokines, which are unleased to create swelling in order to allow for the permeability of nutrients and immune cells in and out of the area. Inflammation results in redness, heat, pain and swelling.

There are three cascading and inter-related systems, which are the source of these chemical mediators that are responsible for the acute inflammatory response: the kinin system, the complement system, and the coagulation system.

The *kinin system* uses a chemical messenger called bradykinin. The activation of bradykinin increases smooth muscle contraction, pain sensation, vascular permeability (passage of nutrients), and vasodilation (expanding of vessels). Bradykinin also plays a role in blood pressure control during inflammatory reactions by actively opening blood vessels, which in turn decreases blood pressure. This means the antagonal pathway acts to increase blood pressure via the hormone signal angiotensin. The popular class of drugs known as ACE inhibitors block the breakdown of bradykinin in order to keep the vessels open to decrease systematic blood pressure in cardiovascular issues.[4] Over time, high pressure throughout the vasculature becomes a chronic stress to the cells lining the arteries, thus leading to injury. This sets the precipice for heart disease, which can be accelerated when combined with other risk factors. The plaque and inflammation found in heart disease is the result of the overall immune system's attempt to repair an injury.

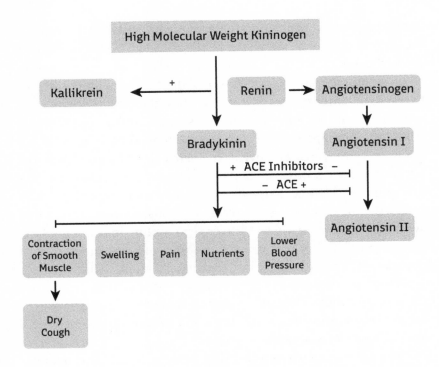

The *complement system* is activated to attack bacteria through opsonization, which is the process by which pathogens are marked down to be destroyed Pac-Man style by phagocytes. Once phagocytes see that an antigen is marked with a red flag they digest it.

The complement system has three potential pathways for opsonization: the antigen-antibody reaction, bacterial endotoxin pathway, and the lectin mannose-binding pathway.

The antigen-antibody reaction occurs when a complement protein binds directly to a foreign antigen. The antigen-antibody pathway can also be activated during adaptive immunity. Once a few proteins attach, they activate enzymes to break down the foreign body. In the bacterial endotoxin pathway, a complement protein will bind to toxins produced by the bacteria. In the lectin mannose pathway, a protein-carbohydrate structure is used to bind to bacteria and viruses. Each pathway follows an order of operations to create specific enzymes and chemical mediators to drive the destruction of the foreign body through an inflammatory process.

The pathways also generally go after different classes of pathogens. Each of the complement protein structures are responsible for attracting different types of adaptive immune cells to the scene that have more specific roles.[5]

The *coagulation system* starts at the level of the cell membrane, where a phospholipid (fatty acid) is produced into arachidonic acid (omega 6 fatty acid). Arachidonic acid is a fatty-acid derivative that stimulates the inflammatory cascade.[6]

Corticosteroid drugs inhibit the phospholipase A2 enzyme, preventing the freeing of arachidonic acid and thereby relieving symptoms of pain and inflammation.[7] Once arachidonic acid is activated it can go down two pathways: COX (cyclooxygenase) and/or LOX (lipoxygenase).

The cyclooxygenase or COX enzyme forms thromboxane and prostaglandins from arachidonic acid. Thromboxane stimulates platelet aggregation and vasoconstriction. Prostaglandins have effects like increasing pain sensation, immunosuppression, vascular spasm, and inhibiting gastric acid secretion. NSAIDs, aspirin,[8] turmeric,[9] and ginger[10] can be used to inhibit the COX enzyme. Pharmacological and nutraceutical agents always affect more than one pathway, so while in addition to getting some desired outcomes, side effects can also arise. For example, NSAIDs decrease inflammation, but also can cause severe damage to the gut lining. Furthermore, when aspirin blocks the COX enzyme it opens the gates for arachidonic acid to be converted to LOX pathway, greatly increasing asthma symptoms. The LOX pathway stimulates smooth muscle contraction, vascular permeability, and chemotaxis of neutrophils, monocytes, and macrophages.[11] This pathway can be inhibited with the drug Zileuton[12] or with the herbs Boswellia (frankincense)[13] and turmeric.

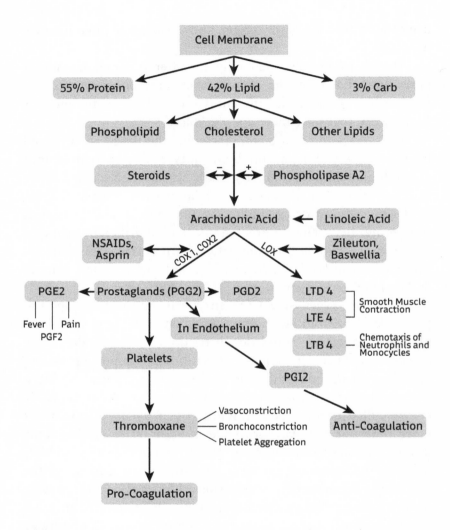

When tissue injury occurs (infection, trauma, autoimmunity), there is a brief transient vasoconstriction of the area followed by a temporary platelet plug, which is created until the coagulation cascade stimulates the platelets to release TXA2 (thromboxane), which forms a stronger fibrin mesh web.[14] This is meant to be effective for the acute healing process.

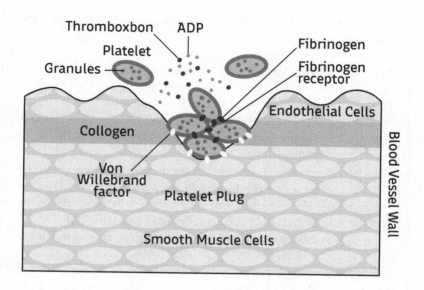

After the rapid constriction of vessels around the area, it then goes directly into dilation, allowing nutrients, platelets, and white blood cells to swell to the area. The white blood cell's role is to neutralize pathogens. While binding and interacting with the pathogens, white blood cells release chemical messengers to either keep inflammation on or turn it off.

The heat and increased blood flow associated with acute inflammation increase the rate of healing. White blood cells are immune fighting cells and release chemical messengers called cytokines. Interleukins are a type of cytokine and are abbreviated as IL with an associated number. Different types of autoimmune disease are associated with a surplus or deficiency in particular cytokines.[15] For example, Irritable Bowel disease is associated with a deficiency in IL-10 to decrease gut inflammation and a surplus of TNF and IL-6.

Following are a few examples of the instructions the chemical messengers code for:

IL-1	Stimulates T cells, inflammation, and fever.
IL-5	Stimulates production of eosinophils.
IL-6	Stimulates B cells and increased production of platelets.
IL-7	Increases production of lymphocytes.
TNF	Signals macrophages, "master regulator" of inflammatory cytokine production, and stimulates cell death.
IL-10	Inhibits inflammation and stimulates production of antibodies.

The Cytokine Network

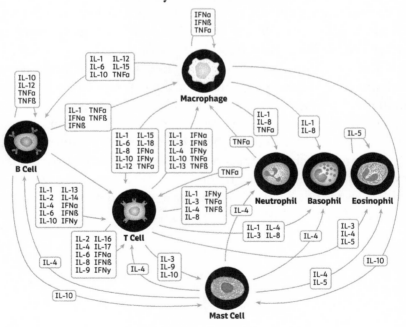

The Cytokine Network diagram illustrates the complex orchestrating of metabolic and immune communications. Interactions with the environment can throw the immune function out of homeostasis, causing a dominance in inflammatory messages.

During an inflammatory event, levels of oxidative stress in the body increase. Oxidative stress refers to an accumulation in reactive oxygen species that are formed during normal metabolism. However, reactive oxygen species are produced in higher amounts due to exposure to heavy metals, toxins, radiation, drugs, and pollutants. They are highly reactive with the cells and organelles in the body and cause DNA and mitochondrial damage.[16] Over time, high levels of oxidation are going to accelerate the aging process and set fertile ground for disease—specifically, for autoimmune disease. Antioxidants and free radical scavengers act to clean up the free radicals. There are ways to both eliminate the creation of excess free radicals and boost free radical scavenging to aid your body in the housekeeping of free radicals. If a balance is not kept, a dominance of oxidants over antioxidants results in disease.

The body is designed to deal with acute stress, and actually benefits from acute stressors like exercise. With that being said, the poison is in the dosage. Too strong an acute stress could also trigger autoimmunity, such as when someone on a night out decides to abuse their body by chain-smoking and washing down beers with immune reactive foods while listening to deafening loud music in the heat, after which they get only a few hours of sleep.

When acute stress lags it can become chronic. Chronic stress results in chronic inflammation over weeks and months leading to tissue destruction. The result of chronic inflammation is immune dysregulation. The body mounts persistent immune cascades that are never given messages to turn off. After all, the immune system is behaving in a way it was designed to, but our bodies are fed environmental signals that we were never meant to sustain. Chronic stress is an amalgamation of diet, toxins, psychological state, infection, radiation exposure, medications, and other factors that appear later in the book. Everybody's body deals with chronic stress in different ways. One person's immune system dysregulation may trigger the body to attack the joints, while another may sustain an attack to the stomach lining, and yet another results in a dermatitis.

White blood cells are responsible for fighting the bad guys. They protect against infections from bacteria, fungi, protozoa, viruses, and parasites. There are many different types of white blood cells, all with their own roles and responsibilities. They circulate the body in the blood and are stored in organs like the thymus, spleen, bone marrow, and lymph nodes.

Organs that house white blood cells

Thymus	T cells mature in the thymus, a small organ found in upper chest. One of the roles of the thymus is to test for auto-activity T cells and destroy them. However, the thymus shrinks as we age, and in the elderly it only works between 1 to 5 percent of the activity it does in children. In studies on animals where the thymus is removed, autoimmunity becomes inevitable.
Bone Marrow	Bone marrow is found within the lumen of long bones. It contains stem cells that can form many different types of cells including immune cells such as neutrophils, eosinophils, basophils, mast cells, monocytes, dendritic cells, and macrophages.
Spleen	This organ is located behind the stomach. Immune cells mature here; upon recognizing blood-borne pathogens, they will activate. The spleen functions as a reservoir for monocytes.

Lymphatic System	The lymphatic system is a network of vessels and tissues made up of lymph (a type of fluid) and lymphoid nodes (lymph organs). It is used as a detoxification and communication network for immune cells. If adaptive immunity is activated, lymph nodes may swell as an indicator of infection. Stem cells can also originate from the lymph system and are largely responsible for the creation of natural killer cells, as well as memory B and T cells.[17]

Organs of the Immune System

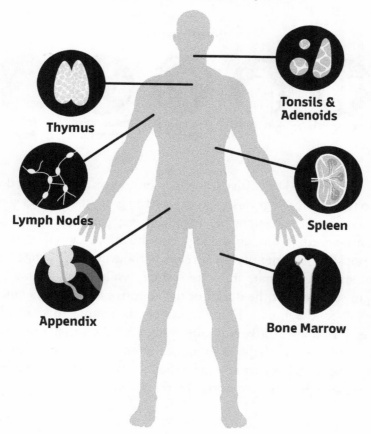

Autoimmune Disease

Heredity **White Blood Cells** **Lifestyle** **Hormone Influence** **Environmental Factors**

  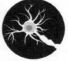

Systemic Lupus Erythematosus **Rheumatoid Arthritis** **Multiple Sclerosis**

Symptoms

Myocarditis **Skin Rash** **Impaired Vision** **Pulmonary Fibrosis** **Joint Pain**

White blood cells, also known as leukocytes, are broken down into two main categories: phagocytes and lymphocytes. As stated, phagocytes are responsible for digesting pathogens that have been marked as foreign through opsonization. Lymphocytes are responsible for identifying foreign pathogenic cells. Phagocytes are part of the innate immune system, while some lymphocytes begin to carry out the duties of the adaptive immune system.

When the innate immune system is unable to control an infection, the adaptive immune system is called to action. There are two types of adaptive immune system: the humoral immune response, which is carried out by the B-cells; and the cell-mediated response, which is carried out by the T-cells.

Types of Phagocytes

Neutrophils	The most common white blood cell, neutrophils are responsible for producing pus to kill invading bacteria, fungi, and protozoa. They play the largest role in bacterial infections. They are activated by Platelet activating factor (PAF).[18, 19]
Monocytes	Monocytes are derived from bone marrow and circulate in the blood and spleen. They have the ability to recognize pathogens via pattern recognition receptors. Monocytes can phagocytize, secrete chemokines, and proliferate in response to infection or injury. They upregulate inflammatory signals such as nitric oxide and secrete pro-inflammatory cytokines.[20]
Mast cells	Responsible for regulating vasodilation, vascular homeostasis, innate and adaptive immune responses, angiogenesis, and poison detoxification. Mast cells play a role in allergies, asthma, anaphylaxis, and gastrointestinal disorders. They release inflammatory mediators such as heparin, histamine, and cytokines. They serve as a first line of defense against antigens entering the body and are located in the skin and mucosa.[21]
Basophils	The least abundant of the leukocytes, basophils play a role in hypersensitivity and inflammatory reactions, including in allergic dermatitis, atopic dermatitis, allergic reactions, anaphylaxis, asthma, Lupus, and Crohn's disease.[22, 23]

Eosinophil	Eosinophils are involved in hosting defense against parasites, promoting allergic reactions, and asthma, and regulating the immune system through cytokines.[24]

On blood panels, if any of these phagocytes are out of range, it helps paint the picture of the type of pathogen the body is fighting.

Types of Lymphocytes

B-Lymphocytes (B cells)	B-lymphocytes produce antibodies or immunoglobulins. The B-lymphocyte cells exist in a resting state until their receptors match with an antigen and quickly start replicating that particular antibody. B-lymphocytes mature in the bone marrow. They can mature into either memory B cells or plasma cells. B cells can have over 100,000 identification and communication receptors on their cell membranes. These are the ultimate reconnaissance units.[25]
T-lymphocytes (T cells)	T-lymphocytes produce immune responses to invaders and eliminate dysfunctional human cells. T-lymphocytes are the major player in autoimmune disease. The tradeoff of producing thousands and thousands of antigen receptors needed to recognize a wide spectrum of pathogens is the risk of producing self-reactive lymphocytes that can trigger autoimmunity. T-lymphocytes mature in the thymus.

Types of T cells

Regulatory T cells	The role of the T cell is telling self from non-self. T-regulatory cells turn off active T cells, thereby preventing autoimmunity. In experiments the removal of T-regulatory cells caused autoimmunity. They are especially abundant in the gut to distinguish between germs and food or friendly bacteria. Before entering the blood stream each B and T cell is tested to see if it reacts to healthy cells in which case it will be destroyed.[26, 27]
Helper T cells	Helper T cells turn on signals when they identify foreign pathogens and secrete cytokine messages that activate B cells to produce antibodies and activate cytotoxic T cells to target pathogens. Helper T cells turn into Th1 and Th2 cells. When Th1 and Th2 cells fall out of ratio or are overproduced, autoimmune disease can manifest.[28]
Cytotoxic T cells	They recognize viral peptides on the surface of cells and then engage and kill the virus and infected cell. Cytotoxic T cells also play a role in eliminating cancer cells. They reserve the ability to inactivate themselves to prevent autoimmunity.[29]
Natural Killer T cells	Natural Killer T cells bridge the adaptive immune system with the innate immune system. They are responsible for fighting microbial infections as well as tumors. Natural killer T cells have the ability to recognize self and non-self, and to heavily secrete Th1 and Th2 cytokines, induce cytotoxicity, and stimulate phagocytes.[30]

| Dendritic cells | Dendritic cells mature from phagocytes, not lymphocytes. Dendritic cells act as messengers between the innate and adaptive immunity. They will preserve peptides broken down by phagocytes and present the antigen on the cell surface of T cells to activate them. Dendritic cells do this by traveling to lymphoid organs to display the peptides from the broken down antigens on their membranes in order for T cells to decide whether to attack antigens with those same peptides. They can also turn off self-reactive T cells by summoning T-regulator cells. Dendritic cells play a role in decreasing immune activity and inflammation.[31] |

Types of B cells

| Memory B cells | Memory B-cells can survive for decades with memory of past antigens. Memory B-cells have the antigen peptide on their surface so that the antigen can be identified when they come in contact. These play an integral role in preventing future infections.[32] |
| Plasma cells | Plasma cells are antibody factories and manufacture antibodies in mass.[33] |

The B- and T-lymphocytes behave under certain checks and balances. B-cells don't get fully activated when they first bind to an antigen as a protective measure. Many of the antigen receptors are created randomly, so it's possible that a receptor is created against a healthy body cell. Let's say it produces a receptor that recognizes your thyroid, without the checks and balances the B-cell would immediately sound the alarm on your thyroid tissue. However, the B cell needs to be activated by Helper T or Regulatory T cells before it is able to take action. Properly functioning Regulatory T cells will not activate autoantibody B cells against healthy cells. Although B cells are the cells that produce autoimmune antibodies, it is incumbent to foster healthy T cell function to prevent autoimmune disease.[34] There will be times when autoantibodies slip through the checks and balances. The numbers are slim and should not be cause for a significant problem within a properly functional immune system.

B-lymphocytes produce five main categories of immunoglobulin or antibody molecules into the serum: IgG, IgM, IgA, IgE, and IgD. They are distinguished by the type of structural bond within its chemical makeup. The variation in chain polypeptides allows each immunoglobulin class to function in a different type of immune response or during a different stage of the body's defense. The antibodies or immunoglobulins lock onto the antigen, flagging it with a chemical so the white blood cells know to attack it and effectively eliminate it.

IgG	IgG are found in body fluids including in blood, lymph fluid, and cerebrospinal fluid.
	IgG can also cross the placenta from the mother into the fetus.
	IgG molecules can react with receptors that are present on the surface of macrophages, neutrophils, and natural killer cells, and they can activate the complement system. This is most important in fighting viral and bacterial infections.
	IgG antibodies tend to be hyperactive in autoimmune disease against our organs and harmless environment antigens.
	IgG antibodies are often neglected on allergy tests.
	IgG stimulate inflammation and the attraction of white blood cells.
	Symptoms of high levels of IgG antibodies are associated with gastrointestinal symptoms, headaches, joint aches, rashes, and autoimmune disease.[35, 36]
IgM	IgM are the first antibodies built during an immune response. They are primarily found in lymph and blood.[37]
IgA	IgA is secreted in breast milk and is also the most prevalent in secretions such as tears, saliva, mucous, and gastric juices, and appears in secretions of ears and the vagina.
	IgA is resistant to digestion and can activate the complement pathway. It is found in the airway and in the digestive tract.
	IgA fights off viral and bacterial infection.[38]

IgE	IgE primarily defends against parasitic invasion and is responsible for allergic reactions. These are the antibodies checked when you go get skin pricked by your allergist.
	IgE react primarily with eosinophils, mast cells, basophils, and histamine release.
	When antigens such as pollen, poisons, fungus, spores, dust mites, or pet dander bind with IgE, it releases factors like proteolytic enzymes, leukotrienes, and cytokines. The typical allergic reactions produce mucus secretion through sneezing, coughing, or tears. These reactions are considered beneficial to rid the body of remaining allergens.[39]
	Symptoms of high levels of IgE antibodies include hives, itchiness, sneezing, teary eyes, shortness of breath, stomach cramps, anaphylaxis, and hay fever.
IgD	Found in the tonsils, spleen, and the linings of cavities such as nasal, lacrimal, salivary, bronchial, and lungs. IgDs play a big role in stimulating inflammation.[40]

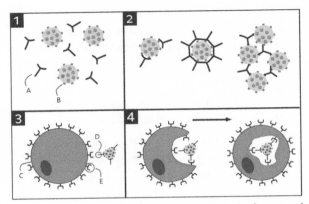

*Antibodies (1A) mark down foreign antigens (1B), dysfunctional cells, or
healthy normal cells as enemy. Macrophages (3C) recognize antibody
receptor (3D) and digest it down (4).*

T-lymphocytes that mature into Helper T cells, can mature
yet again into T-Helper 1 (Th1) or T-Helper 2 cells (Th2). In
homeostasis, a balance of Th1 to Th2 cells are produced. The
two subgroups produce different types of cytokines. When they
become unbalanced, high levels of certain cytokines drive chronic
inflammation, followed by white blood cells and tissue destruction.

Th1 cells are involved in the cell-mediated response and
mount a defense against viruses and bacteria. When Th1 is too
dominant, it plays a role in inflammation and organ specific
autoimmune disease. Th1 is generally involved in delayed
hypersensitive symptoms. Th2 cells are involved in the humoral-
mediated response, which responds to parasites, toxins, and
allergens. When Th2 is too dominant it can play a role in
systematic autoimmune disease. In the cavities, Th1 stimulates
macrophages to eat, while Th2 stimulates secretion of mucus.
Th1 and Th2 are not mutually exclusive and work in conjunction.
For example, Th1 is the red swelling around a mosquito bite, and
the Th2 response is the red bump of the bite.[41] Th1 and Th2 are
not the only T-helper subtypes that play a role in the response,
but not as much is known of these others such as Th17. It is also
theorized that an autoimmune disease can start with a Th1 or
Th2 dominance and then switch as the disease progressives.

Here are some examples of the most common patterns of autoimmune disease.

Th1 Dominant Autoimmunity
Type 1 diabetes[42]
Multiple Sclerosis[43]
Hashimoto's Thyroiditis[44]
Crohn's disease[45]
Rosacea[46]
Psoriasis[47]
Celiac disease[48]
Rheumatoid Arthritis[49]
Vitiligo[50]

Th2 Dominant Autoimmunity
Lupus[51]
Sjogren's Syndrome[52]
Allergic Dermatitis[53]
Eczema[54]
Asthma[55]

| Grave's disease[56] |
| Ulcerative colitis[57] |
| Hypersensitivities (environmental, chemical) |

The complexity of the immune system allows for many different types of dysfunctions to arise. The immune system can become hyperactive and cause autoimmune disease and hypersensitivities as mentioned; however, the immune system can also become underactive and breed immunodeficiency. Immunodeficiencies occur when the immune system has been compromised, thereby exposing the body to infection. It can also be caused by autoimmune diseases that attack immune cells. In a way, cancer can be thought as the opposite of autoimmune disease because it's a hiccup in the immune system's ability to distinguish healthy cells from dysfunctional cells. However, rather than marking down healthy cells as dysfunctional, the immune system fails to mark down dysfunctional cells as such. Immunodeficiencies can be predisposed through genetic mutations or come secondarily from environmental factors, infections, malnutrition, or certain medical treatments such as chemotherapy. Various immunodeficiency disorders can occur from faults in the innate immune system, adaptive system, T-cells, and B-cells. There are over 400 primary immunodeficiencies recognized by the International Union of Immunological Societies.[58]

Hypersensitivities occur when the immune system exaggerates a response against an "antigen" or "allergy." Hypersensitivities are inflammatory immune responses that are harmful to the host and provide a path for autoimmune disease. There are four main pathways of immune hypersensitivities:

Type 1 Immediate Type	IgE binds to "allergen." IgE binds to mast cells and basophils, which then release vasoactive mediators such as histamine, leukotrienes, chemotaxic factors, causing the acute inflammatory cascade. Can become chronic leading to muscular hypertrophy in smooth muscle such as bronchial airways. This is how the body reacts to true allergies (food, animal bites, drugs). It can manifest as asthma, allergies, skin reactions, or shock.[59]
Type 2 cytotoxic-mediated response	IgG and IgM respond against the cell surfaces of our own body cells and extracellular matrix proteins by activating the complement system and stimulating macrophages/neutrophils to the scene. An example of a non-autoimmune Type 2 response is blood transfusion incompatibility. Autoimmune examples include Goodpasture's disease, Grave's disease, Myasthenia Gravis, Type 1 Diabetes, and Hashimoto's thyroiditis.[60]

Type 3 immune complex	Also mediated by IgM and IgG that react with antigens to form antigen-antibody complexes, Type 3 immune complexes slip into circulation (built of toxins, heavy metals, pesticides, etc.) and are unable to be broken down because they are too big, and can thus end up in various tissues and lead to accumulation. Preferred areas of deposition can be the skin, kidney, or joints. The complement system activates and releases cytokines to cause inflammation and tissue damage. Non-Autoimmune examples: mononucleosis, malaria. Autoimmune Examples: Lupus, Rheumatoid Arthritis.[61]
Type 4 delayed type	Caused by direct damage to cells by bacteria, fungi, and viruses, Type 4 delayed type can lead to the formation of granulomas. Non-autoimmune examples: Poison ivy, tuberculosis, schistosomiasis. Autoimmune examples: Sarcoidosis, Crohn's disease. Reaction happens 24–48 hours after exposure to antigen. If caused by a bacteria, the response will usually be Th1.[62]

Is lifestyle causing your glands and cells to misbehave, hyperexcrete, and produce lousy signals? Is your diet damaging the gut lining leading to hypersensitivities? Is the absence of micronutrients inhibiting acceptable immune function? Perhaps, in some cases of autoimmunity, the immune system is responding as it was designed to: to destroy dysfunctional cells. The dysfunctional cells are a result of the chemical signals we are feeding our bodies from the environment. Compounded stress from diet, environment, sun, exercise, psychological problem, noise, or infection can mess with T cell signaling and roll out the red carpet for autoimmune disease in the cascades described in this chapter. When you change your lifestyle and provide the body with new signals and your cells begin to function properly again, the immune system will follow suit. Our goal needs to be to promote normal healthy functioning T cell activity. The reason why the common answer to what causes autoimmune disease is "no one knows" is because it's not a single factor. You can't set up an experiment in humans and introduce one factor and hold everything else constant. However, we can look at animal and epidemiology studies, look at factors that cause inflammation, seek triggers of abnormal changes in immune function, and study clinical case reports. When you decrease chronic oxidative stress, symptoms of autoimmune disease begin to diminish.[63] The tricky part can be uncovering the culprit of stress on the body.

It is not all or nothing either, as autoimmune disease exists on a spectrum kind of like Type II Diabetes. In Diabetes, blood sugar keeps on rising until eventually it has severe consequences, and symptoms arise as it crosses over the threshold to be classified as Diabetes. However, insulin resistance started long before it reached that manmade classification. Markers for autoimmune disease and inflammation also rise this way. You can begin to see positive changes in objective and subjective measures gradually.

A lot of what we know about the immune system has not been around very long. We must remember it is constantly changing thanks to new discoveries. In fact, before the 1950s, autoimmune disease was denied by scientists to be an abstract possibility. Twenty to 30 years from now, immunology will look a lot different than it does today. We will have a better understanding of the immune system mechanisms, and we will have better pharmacological agents. However, what won't change is the benefits of living a conscious, holistic lifestyle that closely replicates that of our ancestors.

The manifestations of most diseases have some overlap. Immune dysregulation in childhood results in allergies and asthma, in young adulthood it transforms into autoimmune disease, towards middle age it morphs into cancer and heart disease, and in old age it results in degenerative diseases like Alzheimer's. Throughout the totality of life, low-grade immune dysregulation results in anxiety and depression. An understanding of the innerworkings of the immune system provides the foundational knowledge for understanding how changes in lifestyle will have a positive effect on reversing chronic autoimmune disease.

N O T E S

1   Cooper, M. D. and Adler, M. N. (2026, Feb. 24). *The Evolution of Adaptive Immune Systems.* Cell. https://www.cell.com/fulltext/S0092-8674(06)00152-8.

2   Alberts, B. (1970, Jan. 1). *Innate immunity.* Molecular Biology of the Cell. 4th ed. https://www.ncbi.nlm.nih.gov/books/NBK26846.

3   MT;, C. S. E. S. L. L. G. J. N. B. *Morphological variation and airflow dynamics in the human nose.* American journal of human biology: the official journal of the Human Biology Council. https://pubmed.ncbi.nlm.nih.gov/15495233.

4   Golias, C.; Charalabopoulos, A.; Stagikas, D.; Charalabopoulos, K.; Batistatou, A. (2007, July). *The kinin system--bradykinin: Biological effects and clinical implications. multiple role of the kinin system--bradykinin.* Hippokratia. https://www.ncbi.nlm.nih.gov/pmc/articles/PMC2658795.

5   Noris, M. and Remuzzi, G. (2013, Nov.). *Overview of complement activation and regulation.* Seminars in nephrology. https://www.ncbi.nlm.nih.gov/pmc/articles/PMC3820029.

6   Williams, C. S.; Mann, M.; DuBois, R. N. (2000, Jan. 4). *The role of cyclooxygenases in inflammation, cancer, and development.* Nature News. https://www.nature.com/articles/1203286.

7   P;, H. A. J. L. (n.d.). *The acute inflammatory process, arachidonic acid metabolism and the mode of action of anti-inflammatory drugs.* Equine veterinary journal. Retrieved from https://pubmed.ncbi.nlm.nih.gov/6428879.

8   Qureshi, O. (2021, April 19). *COX inhibitors.* StatPearls [Internet]. Retrieved from https://www.ncbi.nlm.nih.gov/books/NBK549795.

9   CV;, R. *Regulation of Cox and Lox By curcumin.* Advances in experimental medicine and biology. Retrieved from https://pubmed.ncbi.nlm.nih.gov/17569213.

10 van Breemen, R. B.; Tao, Y.; Li, W. (2011, Jan.). *Cyclooxygenase-2 inhibitors in GINGER (Zingiber Officinale).* Fitoterapia. Retrieved from https://www.ncbi.nlm.nih.gov/pmc/articles/PMC3018740.

11 Hedi, H. and Norbert, G. (2004). *5-Lipoxygenase pathway, DENDRITIC cells, and adaptive immunity.* Journal of biomedicine & biotechnology. Retrieved from https://www.ncbi.nlm.nih.gov/pmc/articles/PMC548806.

12 Rossi, A.; Pergola, C.; Koeberle, A.; Hoffmann, M.; Dehm, F.; Bramanti, P.; Cuzzocrea, S.; Werz, O.; Sautebin, L. (2010, Oct.). *The 5-lipoxygenase INHIBITOR, zileuton, suppresses Prostaglandin biosynthesis BY inhibition of arachidonic Acid release in macrophages.* British journal of pharmacology. Retrieved from https://www.ncbi.nlm.nih.gov/pmc/articles/PMC2990155.

13 Siddiqui, M. Z. (2011, May). *Boswellia serrata, a potential ANTIINFLAMMATORY agent: An overview.* Indian journal of pharmaceutical sciences. Retrieved from https://www.ncbi.nlm.nih.gov/pmc/articles/PMC3309643.

14 Weisel, J. W. and Litvinov, R. I. (2017). *Fibrin formation, structure and properties.* Sub-cellular biochemistry. Retrieved Sept. 11, 2021, from https://www.ncbi.nlm.nih.gov/pmc/articles/PMC5536120.

15 Zhang, J. M. and An, J. (2007). *Cytokines, inflammation, and pain.* International anesthesiology clinics. Retrieved from https://www.ncbi.nlm.nih.gov/pmc/articles/PMC2785020.

16 Pizzino, G.; Irrera, N.; Cucinotta, M.; Pallio, G.; Mannino, F.; Arcoraci, V.; Squadrito, F.; Altavilla, D.; Bitto, A. (2017). *Oxidative stress: Harms and benefits for human health.* Oxidative medicine and cellular longevity. Retrieved from https://www.ncbi.nlm.nih.gov/pmc/articles/PMC5551541.

17 U.S. National Library of Medicine. (2020, July 30). *What are the organs of the immune system?* InformedHealth.org [Internet]. Retrieved from https://www.ncbi.nlm.nih.gov/books/NBK279395.

18 Aquino, E. N.; Neves, A. C. D.; Santos, K. C.; Uribe, C. E.; Souza, P. E. N.; Correa, J. R.; Castro, M. S.; Fontes, W. (2016). Proteomic Analysis of Neutrophil Priming by paf. *Protein and Peptide Letters*, 23(2), 142–151. https://doi.org/10.2174/0929866523666151202210604.

19 Malech, H. L.; DeLeo, F. R.; Quinn, M. T. (2014a). The Role of Neutrophils in the Immune System: An Overview. *Methods in Molecular Biology* (Clifton, N.J.), 1124, 3-10. https://doi.org/10./1007/978-1-62703-845-4_1.

20 Chiu, S. and Bharat, A. (2016). Role of Monocytes and Macrophages in Regulating Immune Response Following Lung Transplantation. *Current Opinion in Organ Transplantation*, 21 (3), 239–245. https://doi.org/10.1097/MOT.0000000000000313.

21 Krystel-Whittemore, M.; Dileepan, K. N.; Wood, J. G. (2016). Mast cell: A Multi-Functional Master Cell. *Frontiers in Immunology*, 6, 620. https://doi.org/10.3389/fimmu.2015.00620.

22 Min, B.; Brown, M. A.; LeGros, G. (2012). Understanding the Roles of Basophils: Breaking Dawn. *Immunology*, 135(3), 192–197. https://doi.org/10.1111/j.1365-2567.2011.03530.x.

23 Cromheecke, J. L.; Nguyen, K. T.; Huston, D. P. (2014). Emerging Role of Human Basophil Biology in Health and Disease. *Current Allergy and Asthma Reports,* 14(1), 408. https://doi.org/10./1007/s11882-013-0408-2.

24 Wen, T. and Rothenberg, M.E. (2016). The Regulatory Function of Eosinophils. *Microbiology Spectrum,* 4(5),. https://doi.org/10.1128/microbiolspec.MCHD-0020-2015.

25 Alberts, B.; Johnson, A.; Lewis, J.; Raff, M.; Roberts, K.; Walter, P. (2002). B cells and Antibodies. *Molecular Biology of the Cell.* 4th ed. https://www.ncbi.nlm.nih.gov/books/NBK26884.

26 Vignali, D. A. A.; Collison, L. W.; Workman, C. J. (n.d.). *How regulatory t cells work.* Nature News. Retrieved from https://www.nature.com/articles/nri2343.

27 Wing, K. and Sakaguchi, S. (2009, Dec. 17). *Regulatory t cells exert checks and balances on self tolerance and autoimmunity.* Nature News. Retrieved from https://www.nature.com/articles/ni.1818?message-global=remove.

28 Alberts, B.."Helper T Cells and Lymphocyte Activation," *Molecular Biology of the Cell.* 4th ed., (1970, Jan. 1). Retrieved from https://www.ncbi.nlm.nih.gov/books/NBK26827.

29 "Cytotoxic T Lymphocyte," *Cytotoxic T Lymphocyte - an overview | ScienceDirect Topics.* Retrieved from https://www.sciencedirect.com/topics/medicine-and-dentistry/cytotoxic-t-lymphocyte.

30 Vivier, E.; Tomasello; E.; Baratin, M.; Walzer, T.; Ugolini, S. (2008, April 18). *Functions of natural killer cells.* Nature News. Retrieved from https://www.nature.com/articles/ni1582.

31 *Dendritic cell.* Dendritic Cell—an overview | ScienceDirect Topics. Retrieved from https://www.sciencedirect.com/topics/biochemistry-genetics-and-molecular-biology/dendritic-cell.

32 *Memory B cell—An overview | ScienceDirect topics.* Retrieved from https://www.sciencedirect.com/topics/medicine-and-dentistry/memory-b-cell.

33 *Plasma cell—An overview | ScienceDirect topics.* (n.d.). Retrieved Sept. 12, 2021, from https://www.sciencedirect.com/topics/medicine-and-dentistry/plasma-cell.

34 Wang, P. and Zheng, S. G. (2013). Regulatory T Cells and B Cells: Implication on Autoimmune Diseases. *International Journal of Clinical and Experimental Pathology.* 6(12), 2668–2674.

35 *Immunoglobulin G Antibody—An overiew | sciencedirect topics.* https://www.sciencedirect.com/topics/neuroscience/immunoglobulin-g-antibody.

36 Coucke F. Food Intolerance in Patients with Manifest Autoimmunity. Observational Study. *Autoimmune Rev.* (2018, Nov.) 17(11):1078–1080.

37 *Immunoglobulin M Antibody—An overiew | sciencedirect topics.* https://www.sciencedirect.com/topics/medicine-anddentistry/immunoglobulin-m.

38 Woof, J. M. and Russel, M.W. (2011). Structure and function relationships in IgA. *Mucosal Immunology.* 4(6), 590–597. https://doi.org/10.1038/mi.2011.39.

39 Oettgen, H. C. (2016). Fifty years later: Emerging Functions of IgE Antibodies in Host Defense, Immune Regulation, and Allergic Diseases.

The Journal of Allergy and Clinical Immunology, . 137(6), 1631–1645. https://doi.org/10.1016/j.jaci.2016.04.009.

40 *Immunoglobulin D—An overview | sciencedirect topics. https://www. sciencedirect.com/topics/medicine-and-dentistry/immunoglobulin-d.*

41 Velasquez-Manoff, M. (2013). *An epidemic of absence: A new way of understanding allergies and autoimmune diseases.* Scribner.

42 Szebeni, A.; Schloot, N.; Kecskemeti, V.; Hosszufalusi, N. (2015), Th1 and Th2 cell responses of type 1 diabetes patients and healthy controls to human heat-shock protein 60 peptides AA437-460 and AA394-408. Inflammation research: Offficial Journal of the European Histamine Research Society . . . (et al.), 54(10), 415–419. https://doi.org/10.1007/s00011-005-1362-9.

43 Lovett-Racke, A. E.; Yang, Y.; Racke, m. K. (2011). Th1 versus Th17: are T cell cytokines relevant in multiple sclerosis? *Biochimica et Biophysica Acta* (BBA)- *Molecular Basis of Disease,* 1812(2), 246–251. https://doi. org/10.1016/j.bbadis.2010.05.012.

44 Phenekos, C.; Vryonidou, A.; Gritzapis, A.D.; (2004). Th1 and Th2 serum cytokine profiles characterize patients with Hoshimoto's thyroiditis (Th1) and Graves' disease (Th2). *Neuroimmunomodulation,.* 11(4), 209–213. https://doi.org/10.1159/000078438.

45 Bentz, S., et. al. Clinical relevance of IgG Antibodies Against Food Antigens in Crohn's Disease: a Double-Blind Cross-over Diet Intervention Study. *Digestion.* 2010. 81(4):252–64.

46 Schlaak, J. F.; Buslau, M.; Jochum, W.; Hermann, E.; Girndt, M.; Gallati, H.; Meyer zum Büschenfelde, K. H.; Fleischer, B. (1994). T cells involved in psoriasis vulgaris belong to the Th1 subset. *The Journal of Investigative Dermatology,* 102(2), 145–149. https://doi.org/10.1111/1523-1747. ep12371752.

47 Schlaak, J. F., et al. (1994). T cells involved in psoriasis vulgaris belong to the Th1 subset. *The Journal of Investigative Dermatology,* . 102(2), 145–149. https://doi.org/10.1111/1523-1747.ep12371752.

48 Holtmann, M. H. and Neurath, M. F. (2004). T helper cell polarisation in coeliac disease: Any (T-)bet ? *Gut,* 53(8), 1065–1067. https://doi. org/10.1136/gut.2003.038232.

49 Schulze-Koops, H. and Kalden, J. R. (2001). The balance of Th1/Th2 cytokines in rheumatoid arthritis. *Best Practice & Research. Clinical Rheumatology,* . 15(5), 677–691. https://doi.org/10.1053/berh.2001.0187.

50 Antonelli, A.; Ferrari, S. M.; Fallahi, P. (2015). The role of the Th1 chemokine CXCL10 in vitiligo. *Annals of Translational Medicine,* 3(Suppl 1), S16. https://doi.org/10.3978/j.issn.2305-5839.2015.03.02.

51 Ishida, H.; Ota, H.; Yanagida, H.; Dobashi, H. (1997). [An imbalance between Th1 and Th2-like cytokines in patients with autoimmune diseases—Differential diagnosis between Th1 dominant autoimmune diseases and Th2 dominant autoimmune diseases]. *Nihon Rinsho. Japanese Journal of Clinical Medicine,* 55(6), 1438–1443.

52   Ishida, H., et al. (1997). [An imbalance between Th1 and Th2-like cytokines in patients with autoimmune diseases—Differential diagnosis between Th1 dominant autoimmune diseases and Th2 dominant autoimmune diseases]. *Nihon Rinsho. Japanese Journal of Clinical Medicine, 55*(6), 1438–1443.

53   Maggi, E. (1998). The TH1/TH2 paradigm in allergy. *Immunotechnology, 3*(4), 233–244. https://doi.org/10.1016/S1380-2933(97)10005-7.

54   Abrahamsson, T. R.; Abelius, M. S.; Forsberg, A.; Björkstén, B.; Jenmalm, M. C. (2011). A Th1/Th2-associated chemokine imbalance during infancy in children developing eczema, wheeze and sensitization. *Clinical & Experimental Allergy, 41*(12), 1729–1739. https://doi.org/10.1111/j.1365-2222.2011.03827.x.

55   Abrahamsson, T. R., et al. (2011). A Th1/Th2-associated chemokine imbalance during infancy in children developing eczema, wheeze and sensitization. *Clinical & Experimental Allergy, 41*(12), 1729–1739. https://doi.org/10.1111/j.1365-2222.2011.03827.x.

56   Phenekos, C.; Vryonidou, A.; Gritzapis, A. D.; Baxevanis, C. N.; Goula, M.; Papamichail, M. (2004). Th1 and Th2 serum cytokine profiles characterize patients with Hashimoto's thyroiditis (Th1) and Graves' disease (Th2). *Neuroimmunomodulation, 11*(4), 209–213. https://doi.org/10.1159/000078438.

57   Bamias, G. and Cominelli, F. (2015). Role of Th2 immunity in intestinal inflammation. *Current Opinion in Gastroenterology, 31*(6), 471–476. https://doi.org/10.1097/MOG.0000000000000212.

58   *Specific Diagnoses | Immune Deficiency Foundation.* Retrieved from https://primaryimmune.org/specific-pi-diagnoses.

59   *Type I Hypersensitivity—An overview | sciencedirect topics.* Retrieved 2021 from https://www.sciencedirect.com/topics/immunology-and-microbiology/type-i-hypersensitivity.

60   Type II Hypersensitvity—An overview / sciencedirect topics. https://www.sciencedirect.com/topics/medicine-and-dentistry/type-ii-hypersensitivity.

61   Type III Hypersensitvity—An overview / sciencedirect topics. https://www.sciencedirect.com/topics/medicine-and-dentistry/type-iii-hypersensitivity.

62   Type IV Hypersensitvity—An overview / sciencedirect topics. https://www.sciencedirect.com/topics/medicine-and-dentistry/type-iv-hypersensitivity.

63   *The influence of reactive oxygen species in the immune system and pathogenesis of multiple sclerosis.* https://read.qxmd.com/read/32789026/the-influence-of-reactice-oxygen-species-in-the-immune-system-and-pathogenesis-of-multiple-sclerosis?sid=48b73760-4d08-4736-8376-2c5a9b2c4d96.

CHAPTER 2

Conventional Medicine

ANY PEOPLE READING THIS CHAPTER have already been through the wringer of pharmaceutical drugs and may not have responded or, worse, have experienced side effects. It is important to understand the conventional approach to treating autoimmune disease and why it is not the superior long-term solution in eliminating symptoms, optimizing quality of life, and becoming the best version of yourself. There is value in conventional diagnostics for measuring markers of autoimmune disease and tracking them over time.

I wish we could just take a magic pill and all our problems would go away. However, there is no such thing as a free metabolic lunch. If you take a pill to inhibit one pathway it opens up the gates to activation and inhibition of pathways you don't want altered. With that being said, pharmaceuticals can have profound effects and you should find a physician who is open-minded to the approach taken in the Kash Code, while also taking a conservative approach with pharmaceutical agents. It is important if you are currently on medications to continue, and as symptoms subside, you can have the conversation with your prescribing doctor to begin to wean off of them. As your symptoms improve, markers of autoimmune disease will also begin to disappear. From a clinical testing perspective, some may be curious as to what classifies them into being placed into a labeled autoimmune disease. This begins with a look at the specific inflammatory markers and antibodies associated with the disease classification.

The first set of drugs commonly prescribed are nonsteroidal anti-inflammatories (NSAIDs) and corticosteroids. NSAIDs act to decrease inflammation and pain associated with autoimmune disease. Nonselective NSAIDs inhibit both Cox-1 and Cox-2 pathways. Therefore, they inhibit platelet aggregation and can cause significant gastrointestinal disorders such as bleeding and ulcers. The Kash Code aims at doing the exact opposite, to bulletproof gut health. In fact, long-term NSAID use is the number one cause of leaky gut, about which we will go into in more depth in the next chapter. Examples of NSAIDs are aspirin and ibuprofen. There are also more specific COX enzyme inhibitors, which simply inhibit the COX-2 enzyme, resulting in fewer side effects. However, some of the adverse effects of COX-2 inhibitors on the cardiovascular system include: congestive heart failure, acute myocardial fraction, and sudden death. COX-2 selective drugs include celecoxib, valdecoxib, and rofecoxib.

Corticosteroids act to suppress the overacting immune system by inhibiting cellular signaling such as cytokine production. They are very effective at blowing out inflammation and are typically used during autoimmune flareups. Some are designed to have specific local effects, and others nuke the entire body. Although the corticosteroids are very powerful in decreasing inflammation, they also induce severe side effects with long-term usage including: gastrointestinal ulcers and bleeding, infection, immunosuppression, and bone damage. Corticosteroids can be used topically, orally, or injected. Some examples include prednisone, hydrocortisone, and dexamethasone.

The next level of pharmaceutic agents includes disease-modifying antirheumatic drugs (DMARDs). DMARDs also act to interfere with cytokine chemical signaling in the inflammatory cascade. Side effects include serious infections, bruising, bleeding, swelling, cancer, gastrointestinal damage, cirrhosis, and neuropathy. Types of DMARDs include hydroxychloroquine, sulfasalazine, and mesalamine. I was prescribed mesalamine, which ultimately triggered inflammatory arthritis in joints throughout my entire body.

In addition, there are drugs referred to as biologics. Biologics are actually IgG antibodies that are designed to attack the hyperactive cells of your immune system. For example, an anti-TNF biologic blocks and binds TNF from transmitting its message. TNF is the ringleader in the inflammatory cascade. It is secreted from inflamed cells and has the ability to induce cell death to prevent the proliferation of a tumor. This was one medication I had some success with; however, it caused me to catch colds/coughs quite frequently. Many patients won't have any response to anti-TNF therapy. Side effects of biologics include increased risk of cancer, triggering of other autoimmune diseases, worsening of autoimmunity, infection, nervous system disorders, birth defects, depression, heart failure, and more. Types of biologics include Humira, Kineret, and Entyvio.[1]

Other drugs used to mask the symptoms of autoimmune disease include proton pump inhibitors (PPIs), selective serotonin reuptake inhibitors (SSRIs), and antihistamines. Heartburn is a symptom associated with gut problems and the failure of the lower esophageal sphincter to close causes back flow of stomach acid into the esophagus. Proton pump inhibitors act by inhibiting the production of stomach acid. Chest pain may temporarily go away, but it is likely to cause long term problems. Decreasing stomach acid allows for bacteria to survive the stomach environment, leading to overgrowth of bad bacteria in the intestines. Furthermore, failure of the lower esophageal sphincter to close is usually caused by a deficit in stomach acid. Stomach acid gives the reflex for the lower esophageal sphincter to close. Diet is the biggest driver in heartburn. Other side effects of PPIs are headaches, nausea, diarrhea, infection, and dependence.[2]

Due to the gut-brain axis, inflammation in the gut can cause inflammation in the brain, which can lead to depression and anxiety. Depression is a symptom often associated with autoimmune disease. Commonly prescribed drugs for depression are SSRIs. They work in a recycling process whereby serotonin is made more available by blocking its reuptake. The effects include insomnia, headaches, rashes, joint pain, reduced sexual desire, and suicidal thoughts.[3] Randomized control trials have found exercise to be just as effective for treating depression as antidepressant medications.[4]

Antihistamines are a class of drugs used to combat symptoms of hypersensitivities such as itching, sneezing, and hives. Histamine in the body is a stress signal and opens pores in vessels to allow blood to swell in for an inflammatory response. In the brain histamine actually has a different signal. In fact, it doesn't increase pore size, but rather stimulates nutrient flow to neurons for growth. Under stress, this signal allows the brain to increase computing power during emergencies. While the human body can bias which tissues receive the histamine signal, antihistamines do not bias which tissues it inhibits. Histamine can activate an H1 response (toxic) or H2 response (growth). So it will in fact decrease allergic reactions. However, it will also downregulate neuronal circulation and inhibit nerve function, thereby creating side effects of drowsiness and confusion.[5]

Antidiuretics are another class of drugs used to cover symptoms of frequent and loose bowel movement. Loperamide is used for the control and symptomatic relief of acute diarrhea and of chronic diarrhea that is associated with Inflammatory Bowel Disease. Loperamide binds to opiate receptors in the gut to decrease intestinal peristalsis (contractions). I used to have to pop antidiuretics like candy to get through the day. Other drugs that are used as antidiuretics include Imodium, diphenoxylate, cholestyramine, and codeine sulfate. Side effects include: drowsiness, stomach pain, dizziness, constipation, and addiction.[6]

Autoimmune markers are important to track as objective measures in the progress leading to the journey back to health. Autoimmune antibody tests are used to help diagnose autoimmune disorders. They are designed to detect and measure the levels of autoantibodies. The levels of antibodies can also be used as markers of the severity of your autoimmune disease. Dwindling numbers of antibodies show that the treatment approach is successful and can be confirmed with your subjective symptoms. Antibodies can appear in the body for over a decade before autoimmune symptoms are felt.[7]

Examples of some autoantibodies found in various autoimmune diseases

Antinuclear Antibody (ANA)	Found in individuals with Lupus, Scleroderma, Sjogren's syndrome, or Polymyositis.
Anti DNA Antibody	Found in individuals with Lupus but can also be present in other autoimmune diseases.
Anti–Smooth Muscle Antibody (ASMA)	Found in individuals with Autoimmune Hepatitis, Ulcerative Colitis, Rheumatoid Arthritis, and Polymyositis.
Rheumatoid Factor (RF)	Found in the blood and joint fluids of individuals who have Rheumatoid Arthritis. People who have other diseases may also have RF in their blood, so RF is not specific for Rheumatoid Arthritis.
Glomerular Basement Membrane Autoantibody (GBMA)	Found in individuals who have Autoimmune Kidney Disorders such as Glomerulonephritis or Lupus.

Antineutrophil-Cytoplasmic Antibody (ANCA)	Found in individuals with Rheumatoid Arthritis, Lupus, or Vasculitis.
Antiphospholipid Antibody (APA)	Found in individuals who have Lupus or Vasculitis.
Islet Cell Antibodies (ICAs)	Found in Type I Diabetes.
Parietal Cell Antibody	Found in individuals with Gastric Autoimmunity.
Intrinsic Factor Antibody	Found in individuals with Pernicious Anemia.
Tropomyosin Antibody	Found in individuals with Autoimmune Cardiovascular disease.
Thyroglobulin Antibody, Thyroid Peroxidase Antibody (TPO)	Found in individuals with Autoimmune Thyroid disease, Hashimoto's, and Grave's disease.
21 Hydroxylase Antibody	Found in individuals with Addison's disease, Adrenal Autoimmunity, Autoimmune Endocrine disorders, Diabetes Insipidus, Grave's Disease, Hashimoto's Thyroiditis, and Vitiligo.
Antimyocardial Antibody	Found in individuals with Autoimmune Myocarditis and Rheumatic Heart disease.
Intrinsic Factor antibody	Found in individuals with Pernicious Anemia.

Collagen Complex	Found in individuals with Goodpasture syndrome and Lupus.
Myelin Basic Protein Antibody	Found in individuals with Multiple Sclerosis, Autism, and Lupus.
Synapsin Antibody	Found in individuals with Multiple Sclerosis.
Glutamic Acid Decarboxylase 65 (GAD 65) Antibody	Found in individuals with Batten disease, Celiac disease, Autoimmune Endocrine Disorder, and Type I Diabetes.[8]

Levels of complement proteins that destroys bacteria could also be measured. They play a role in inflammation. Abnormal levels of complement are used to detect immune dysfunction and diagnose autoimmune disorders.

Immune Complex studies can be performed to diagnose and monitor conditions such as Rheumatoid Arthritis, Lupus, Multiple Sclerosis, and Glomerulonephritis. Immune complexes are formed from antibodies that combine with antigens and travel as a mass. These complexes can damage tissues, organs, and joints. Their relatively large mass can become blocked in vessels and tubules.

Tests can be done to learn about inflammatory signals, cytokine profiles, or lymphocytes maps. Specific inflammatory chemical messengers can be identified along with other inflammatory markers like C-reactive protein test. Markers of systemic inflammation can be a sign of Lupus, Rheumatoid Arthritis, and other autoimmune conditions. Cytokine profiles can also measure for Th1 vs. Th2 dominance to see which signaling molecules are playing a role in your autoimmunity. Immunotype includes testing the characteristics of immune cells such as size, shape, density, and granularity to detect early-stage autoimmune disease. These tests can change the treatment approach.

For gut-related autoimmune disease, immune markers like calprotectin, eosinophil protein x, lactoferricin, lysozyme, and secretory IgA can be tracked during the rehabilitation phase to measure progress.

Pharmaceutical agents come with many risks and little promise for the reversal of autoimmune disease. They can, however, provide short-term relief of symptoms and may aid in calming down inflammation, and can be used initially in conjunction with the Kash Code. Throughout the journey it is pertinent to track markers to see treatment progress, so it can be better customized for you. Technology for tracking markers is becoming more precise and effective.

N O T E S

1   Li, P.; Zheng, Y.; Chen, X. (2017). Drugs for autoimmune inflammatory diseases: From small molecule compounds to anti-tnf biologics. *Frontiers in Pharmacology*, 8, 460. https://doi.org/10.3389/fphar.2017.00460.

2   Jaynes, M. and Kumar, A. B. (2018, Nov. 19). *The risks of long-term use of Proton Pump Inhibitors: A critical review*. Therapeutic advances in drug safety. Retrieved from https://www.ncbi.nlm.nih.gov/pmc/articles/PMC6463334.

3   Ferguson, J. M. (2001). SSRI antidepressant medications: Adverse effects and tolerability. *Primary Care Companion to The Journal of Clinical Psychiatry*, 3(1), 22–27.

4   Cooney GM; Dwan K; Greig CA; Lawlor DA; Rimer J; Waugh FR; McMurdo M; Mead GE; (n.d.). *Exercise for depression. The Cochrane database of systematic reviews*. Retrieved from https://pubmed.ncbi.nlm.nih.gov/24026850/

5   Lipton, B. H.; Bensch, K. G.; Karasek, M. A. (1992). Histamine-modulated transdifferentiation of dermal microvascular endothelial cells. *Experimental Cell Research*, 199(2), 279–291. https://doi.org/10.1016/0014-4827(92)90436-C.

6   *Side effects of imodium (Loperamide hcl), warnings, uses.* (n.d.). RxList. Retrieved from https://www.rxlist.com/imodium-side-effects-drug-center.htm.

7   de Brito Rocha, S.; Baldo, D. C.; Andrade, L. E. C. (2019). Clinical and pathophysiologic relevance of autoantibodies in rheumatoid arthritis. *Advances in Rheumatology*, 59(1), 2. https://doi.org/10.1186/s42358-018-0042-8.

8   *Multiple Autoimmune Reactivity Screen Array 5*. Cyrex Labs. (2021). Retrieved from https://www.cyrexlabs.com/Portals/0/Docs/ClinicalApplications/ClinicalAppArray5.pdf.

CHAPTER 3

The Elimination Diet

"All disease begins in your gut."

—Hippocrates

*T*HE HUMAN DIGESTIVE SYSTEM is designed to absorb as many nutrients and as much energy as possible while eliminating and mitigating the effects of toxins and pathogens. The three main sources of energy are fats, carbohydrates, and protein, all of which are commonly referred to as macronutrients. The vitamins and minerals in these foods are referred to as micronutrients. Digestion seeks to break down these compounds into their smallest and most bioavailable forms. The digestive tract is a hollow tube that selectively allows certain particles in while keeping others out. The tract includes the mouth, pharynx, larynx, stomach, small intestines, and large intestines. Axillary organs such as the tongue, salivary glands, pancreas, liver, and gallbladder are involved in producing enzymes that get mixed into the digestive system. The gut is the greatest source of stress relevant to autoimmune disease. Food intolerances, toxins, nutrient deficiencies, and dysbiosis all contribute to stress signals that blur the immune system's ability to tell self from non-self.

Digestion starts with seeing, smelling, or thinking about food, which stimulates the release of enzymes in the stomach and hormones throughout the body. Simultaneously, this imitation innervates the Vagus nerve (cranial nerve 10), which is responsible for the parasympathetic nervous system ("rest and digest"). As food encounters the surface area of the tongue, if the taste is agreeable, secretions of saliva and mechanical manipulation of the food will ensue. The chemosensory properties of the tongue are protective to insure you don't consume toxic or spoiled foods. The saliva is made up of amylase and lingual lipase to break simple fats and sugars. Humans on average produce 0.5–1.5 L of saliva a day.[1] This softened mix of saliva and food is called a bolus.

Next comes the pharynx, which lies behind the nasal cavity and mouth, but above the larynx and esophagus. The pharynx is a tube for both air and food. Its responsibility is to contract food down. The flap on top of the larynx is called the epiglottis, which closes when you are breathing and opens when swallowing. Upon closure, air enters the trachea to be brought down into the lungs. Occasionally, food will slip into the trachea, giving rise to the expression "it went down the wrong pipe," as a product of a strong coughing reflex. The epiglottis has taste buds on it and serves to prevent food from regurgitating.

The diaphragm separates the thoracic cavity from the abdominal cavity where the digestive organs are held. This muscle attaches to various organs in the digestive system. Proper breathing mechanics include breathing into the stomach rather than into the chest. Belly breathing contracts the diaphragm, thus allowing for better digestion and stimulation of the parasympathetic nervous system.

The esophagus connects into the stomach via the lower esophageal sphincter. The stomach holds high levels of hydrochloric acid (HCL) and sodium chloride. Humans have one of the most acidic stomachs in the animal kingdom, between 1–2 pH, that of scavengers. Impressive carnivores like lions have a pH between 2–3, and herbivores are typically between 5–6.[2]

Gastrin is produced by G cells in the stomach to activate other digestive hormones. Gastric chief cells produce pepsinogen, which activates pepsin when combined with HCL, needed to break down proteins. The mechanical motion of the stomach wall is called peristalsis and acts to increase the mixing of food with gastric enzymes. Eventually, the food makes it to the pyloric sphincter (the gate between the stomach and small intestines), where more enzymes are released. The mixture, now referred to as chyme, moves into the proximal portion of the small intestines, the duodenum, where it mixes with enzymes from the pancreas, liver, and gallbladder. Enteroendocrine cells in the stomach lining release serotonin and histamine, which stimulates blood flow to digestive organs.

The Components of the Digestive System

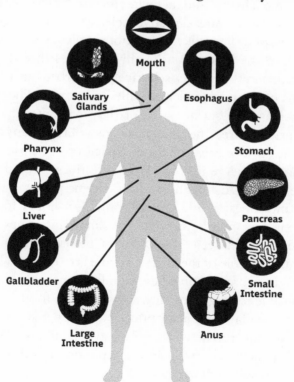

Mouth

Salivary
Glands

Esophagus

Pharynx

Stomach

Liver

Pancreas

Gallbladder

Small
Intestine

Large
Intestine

Anus

In addition to the spleen's role in the immune system, it produces bilirubin, which the liver then converts into bile. Bile is a greenish brown alkaline fluid that plays a role in breaking down fats. Bile is stored in the gallbladder before being released into the small intestines, by the messenger peptide cholecystokinin (CCK). The gallbladder is located directly below the liver.

The pancreas lies behind the stomach. The pancreatic duct attaches to the common bile duct, mixing pancreatic enzymes with bile as it is secreted into the duodenum. Pancreatic enzymes digest proteins and fats. After the food is diffused into the bloodstream, the pancreas produces insulin to encourage cells to absorb the nutrients. The liver produces the hormone glucagon, which stimulates cells to release stored energy into the blood when blood sugars are low.

The small intestine has a higher pH than the stomach to neutralize the chyme and activate incoming enzymes. Lining the small intestines are digestive cells called enterocytes that have microscopic fingerlike projections called villi that absorb nutrients into the blood. As the chyme moves through the rest of the small intestine, it is selectively absorbed into fingerlike projections of the intestinal wall called microvilli. The microvilli greatly increase the surface area of the small intestines by 60–120x.[3] Furthermore, the intestines also have many folds to increase the surface area for food particles to be absorbed. The small intestines merge into the large intestines through a pouch called the cecum. At this intersection chyme passes a valve into the large intestines. While it takes only 6–8 hours for food to travel from the mouth through the small intestines, it takes large intestines between 30–40 hours before having a bowel movement.[4] The role of the large intestine is to absorb water back into the body to prevent diarrhea. Significant numbers of bacteria are responsible for digesting down some of the food to make the vitamins bioavailable for absorption. Normal peristaltic waves of the large intestine run between 5–35 waves a minute.[5] Waves that are too infrequent will result in constipation, and those that are too fast will result in diarrhea.

In the large intestine, food is fermented by gut bacteria. Our large intestines are much smaller than those of our primate cousins. We have lost the ability to ferment plant foods into fat for energy, suggesting our limited ability to break down as much plant roughage. At this point in digestion, the clump is referred to as feces and is pushed along by contractions in the intestinal walls.

In the entire body, 70 to 80 percent of the immune cells are located in the gut,[6] which is like a fortified military fortress where the slightest sign of enemy presence will initiate the alarms. Although the gut is extremely resilient, a lot of problems can arise from our digestive system. NSAIDs, pesticides, herbicides, birth control, sleep deprivation, psychological and physical stress, antibiotic abuse, infections, and processed foods can all play a role in something called leaky gut syndrome.

Throughout your intestines, permeable channels in the wall selectively allow nutrients to enter into the blood stream. Chronic exposure to toxins and stress damage the microvilli and the selective gates, causing them to gap open much larger than they should be. The decreased surface area of the damaged villi prevents needed nutrient absorption. This couples with the widened gates to allow larger molecules, that would not normally be given access, to slip through into the blood stream. Your body can become confused by these foreign proteins and might attack them, leading to allergic reactions or a chronic low-grade immune reaction throughout the body. This can stimulate the immune system to be in a prolonged heightened state birthing autoimmunity. The consumption of copious amounts of artificial food/liquid into your gut every day precisely where there is heavy presence of the immune cells, creates a perfect environment for the brewing of immune dysregulation. This clearly illustrates how food becomes the biggest stress lever in treating autoimmune disease. Leaky gut is associated with Type I Diabetes, Lupus, IBD, Autoimmune Hepatitis, Multiple Sclerosis, and Celiac disease.[7]

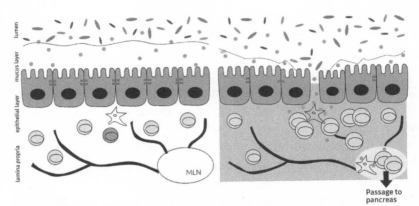

Intact Intestinal Barrier   Compromised Intestinal Barrier

Lipopolysaccharides (LPS) are endotoxins released from the outer membrane of gram-negative bacteria when they die. When the LPS slip through the widened gap junctions, they elicit a uniquely strong immune response from lymphocytes.[8] Often, the binding sites of white blood cells to antigens can be similar to those on human cells in various parts of the body. When an immune response to LPS or food antigens mistakenly stimulates an immune reaction elsewhere in the body, it is referred to as molecular mimicry. A strong immune response to endotoxins can result in white blood cells going after skin, joint, or brain cells. There are many physicians and researchers who believe that leaky gut is a precondition for autoimmune disease. Even in cases where leaky gut does not cause autoimmune disease, it will cause chronic low-grade inflammation, which is the root cause of all chronic diseases.

One method of testing for leaky gut is with the lactulose mannitol test. This test measures levels of these two sugars in a patient's urine after oral ingestion. Mannitol is much smaller in size than lactulose. In a person with a robust gut lining, mannitol is expected to be measured in much larger amounts. A higher lactulose-mannitol ratio implies a greater severity of leaky gut syndrome. Other gut and digestive pathologies that can contribute or cause leaky gut syndrome include: hypochlorhydria (low stomach acid), insufficient digestive enzymes, and small intestinal bacterial overgrowth (SIBO). Many of these gut issues contribute to one another.

Hydrochloric acid (HCL) is needed to break down foods for digestion as well as to kill bacteria on the food. Low stomach acid production can be caused by vitamin deficiencies (zinc, b vitamins),[9, 10] stress, smoking, alcohol abuse, medications, and poor diet. As mentioned in previous chapters, proper amounts of HCL are needed to trigger the reflex of the lower esophageal sphincter to prevent heartburn. Processed, vegetarian, or vegan diets that are low in protein can cause the stomach to produce less HCL. If there is dysfunction at the top of the digestive tract it will cause problems downstream. Low stomach acid leads to an overgrowth in bacteria in the small intestines,[11] causing symptoms of gas and bloating. Additionally, it can place pressure on the lower esophageal sphincter, thus forcing it open.

If stomach pH is too high (less acidic), the chyme will also be as it enters the small intestines, which, in turn, will fail to stimulate pancreatic enzymes responsible for breaking down fats, carbohydrates, and proteins.[12] Undigested food leads to small intestinal bacterial overgrowth (SIBO). Another cause of low stomach acid is being in a chronic state of stress.[13] When the body is in fight-or-flight mode, digestion becomes a second priority; the body does not mobilize its resources to produce stomach acid to digest food. It is important to eat in a relaxed state. Prior to your meal, take a few deep breaths to stimulate the parasympathetic nervous system, and then eat slowly, mindfully, and chew the food until it is in liquid form before swallowing. This will render the nutrients more absorbable and lessen the burden on the digestive system, especially when enzyme levels are low.

Overgrowth of bad bacteria can decrease fat absorption due to bacterial deconjugation of bile salts.[14] Fat absorption, however, is one of the prerequisites for forming bile. Insufficient bile production inhibits the ability to digest fats. Reduced fat absorption hinders absorption of fat-soluble vitamins such as A, D, E, and K. The overgrowth of bacteria can feed on vitamin B12 and iron, inhibiting their absorption.[15] When these micronutrients are deficient in the body, they contribute to immune dysregulation, especially vitamin D. Symptoms that reflect bile deficiency include a metallic taste in the mouth, itchy skin, stools that float, or clay-colored stools.

Gut inflammation from SIBO finances axillary symptoms of autoimmune disease such as depression, anxiety, and mood disorders.[16] SIBO has also been associated with IBD, Scleroderma, and Celiac disease.[17] One study found 100 percent of patients with Fibromyalgia had SIBO.[18] Irritable Bowel Syndrome (IBS) has many of the same symptoms as IBD (constipation, diarrhea, stomach pain). The main differential is the absence of inflammatory markers or degeneration in the walls of the intestines in IBS. IBS is also infamous for being a diagnosis of exclusion, meaning the doctor doesn't know what is causing your gut problems, so they slap the IBS label on it. Certain forms of IBS can be autoimmune because of antibodies that have recently been discovered to play an active role in the syndrome.[19] Today, 15 percent of the U.S. population have IBS,[20] 60 percent experience acid reflux in a given year, and 20 to 30 percent experience reflux on a weekly basis.[21] These gut dysfunctions are extremely common and are a result of diet and lifestyle.

Gut dysfunction leads to altered chemical and immune signaling. Inflammatory cytokines in the gut travel through the blood stream, cross the blood-brain barrier, and then suppress the activity in the frontal cortex of the brain. Like the gut, brain inflammation can cause a leaky blood-brain barrier (BBB), whereby particles can slip in and out of the brain cavity more freely.[22] This can cause the symptoms that are labeled as depression. If that's the case, the solution to some forms of depression is not to provide exogenous neurotransmitters, but rather to restore a healthy gut ecosystem. When activated, the Vagus nerve stimulates digestive activities. Inflammation in the gut can inhibit the parasympathetic input of the Vagus nerve and create a chronic state of fight-or-flight, causing immunodeficiency and further discombobulation within the digestive system. Furthermore, the Vagus nerve can be downregulated at the level of the brain, stimulating inflammation in the gut,[23] which is explained in depth in Chapter 5.

Unfortunately, modern life has disrupted the gut health of most of the population. But there are a few steps that can break the vicious cycle of gut issues. The steps are:

1. **Replace**

   Replace deficient enzymes with substitutes: bile, pancreatic enzymes, HCL, etc.

   With a stool panel, enzymes and HCL can be tested to monitor ranges. Supplementing with enzymes or HCL may initially be warranted until the body is able to begin producing them in sufficient amounts. Proper levels of enzymes are needed to digest foods, kill bacteria, and extract nutrients. This will be further discussed in Chapter 12.

2. **Remove**

   There are several ways to break down and kill the bad bacteria, including the removal of any potential foods that may be triggering the immune system. This is the main focus of this chapter.

3. **Repopulate**

   This includes repopulating the gut with beneficial bacteria while depopulating the bad bacteria. This is explored in the section on the microbiome in Chapter 4.

4. **Repair**

   Providing the right building blocks for the reparation of the gut lining through various supplements, which is addressed in Chapter 12.

Let's now dive into strategies to eliminate food triggers. We must use the power of diet to dial down inflammation. Remember that chronic inflammation causes T cell dysfunction. However, there is no "one size fits all."

The best approach to finding out which foods are triggering immune reactions is to do an elimination diet. A superfood for one individual might actually be highly toxic to another individual. Anyone who suggests one ideal diet that is the optimal for everyone lacks understanding of the personalized approach to nutrition. Sometimes an individual eliminates a particular food or a group of foods, and it has a tremendous positive effect on their condition. This may lead to a mental trap whereby they believe it is the same cure to everyone else's autoimmune disease or health problems.

Most food allergy tests look for IgE antibodies, which are involved in allergic reactions. Allergic reactions are usually immediate and easy to detect. However, many conventional practitioners overlook IgG and IgA antibody testing, which test for food intolerances. These antibodies cause low-grade chronic immune reactions and are harder to uncover as the culprit. In fact, IgG and IgA antibodies could take up to three days to mount their full effects.[24] Although food intolerance tests can give you a more targeted approach to which foods to eliminate, they do not provide 100 percent accuracy.

> *"Nothing in Biology makes sense except in the light of Evolution"*
>
> —Theodosius Dobzhansky

For over 100,000 generations, the human diet varied regionally and seasonally and consisted primarily of wild meat, fish, fruits, vegetables, nuts and seeds. The time period from 2.5 million years ago up until 10,000 years ago is known as the Paleolithic era, hence the "paleo diet."[25] Meat was the most prized and advantageous food for humans to consume during this time period and led to a selective adaptability in our genome to most efficiently acquire it. Our evolution favored adaptations to make us better hunters, including: an upright posture, a unique shoulder joint for throwing, endurance running, sweat glands, and new tendons.[26] These adaptations, combined with the technological advancement of fire and stone tools, set the stage for humans to rise from scavengers to apex predators at the top of the food chain. Climate change, in combination with overhunting of big game like mammoths and other megafauna, forced us into farming at various time points around the globe. This is known as the Neolithic revolution that took place around 10,000–25,000 years ago.[27, 28, 29]

The Neolithic revolution introduced grains, legumes, refined flour, dairy, and domesticated animals. Archaeological evidence from the time of Neolithic revolution indicates that humans became shorter in stature, had increased cases of anemia, experienced a decrease in brain volume and bone density and an increase in infection, bone lesions, cavities, and had higher infant mortality.[30, 31, 32] Then came the Industrial Revolution where white flour, vegetable oil, and table sugar could be mass produced, price reduced, and shipped efficiently. These new foods had much higher calories per gram with fewer nutrients. Fast forward to modern times where these unevolutionary consistent foods have extended into a wider range of rancid oils, processed foods, dyes, additives, fillers, genetically modifying organisms, and artificial foods made in a lab. These unnatural foods, with little to no nutrient value, place tremendous stress on our bodies right where the immune system walks a fine line. The major problem is that these unnatural foods are not rarities, but rather have become staples in the standard American diet.

Contemporary hunter-gatherers who have mostly preserved a paleo era diet live just as long as Western society, but without any of the chronic disease or autoimmune disease.[33] Historically, when roads and highways were built up to native populations, the precipice of modern disease began from the trade of modern foods. As more isolated communities began to consume Western foods, they very quickly inherited our health epidemics. Humans can survive on processed foods, but it is very clear that we do not thrive. In fact, we suffer.

There is not one ideal diet for all humans, as our ancestors came from different regions, and we all inherit different digestive abilities and organ efficiency. Contemporary hunter-gatherers maintain a diverse diet from one another: the Kitavans of Papua New Guinea consume fish, root vegetables, fruits, and coconuts; the Inuit of the Arctic consume over 90 percent of their calories from the saturated fat of seal and whale blubber; and the Aboriginals of Australia live on land mammals, reptiles, insects, and vegetables. Some tribes have adapted genes in the last 10,000 years where the majority of them can break down lactase into adulthood, including the Maasai tribe of Kenya, who consume most their calories from whole raw milk, blood, and beef from their grass-fed cows.[34] Or the Hadza of Tanzania who have increased production of amylase in order to better digest carbohydrates.[35] Even with these diversities of diet, all of these groups have robust health markers, and the absence of modern diseases. Populations that remained as hunter-gatherers for the longest time suffer the most devastation when transferred to a Western diet because of very little genetic adaptability to this modern diet. This is seen in Native Americans who suffer much higher levels of heart disease, diabetes, and various autoimmune disease.[36, 37]

Another major variable is proximity to the equator. Humans who live far from the equator had to endure winters with little access to plant foods or carbohydrates and likely endured long states of ketosis (see Chapter 7 for a detailed explanation), while those who lived close to the equator had year-round access to seasonal plant foods. Ancestrally, environmental discrepancies affected enzyme production, microbiome, and detoxification pathways. Humans have much greater genetic diversity than other animal species because of our far-reaching global presence, which has led to vast adaptations. Some individuals may have longer large intestines for increased ability to digest fibers, while others have longer small intestines and gallbladders for fat digestion. Yet some have an increased number of nerves connecting to digestive organs, and others have differently shaped and sized stomachs that can hold six to eight times more food. This is referred to as biochemical individuality—one's own unique ability to metabolize nutrients with their own set of capabilities.[38] Our genome likely has adapted somewhat in the last 10,000 years, but not fast enough to keep up with environmental changes and food technology.

As illustrated through real world examples, nutrition is very individualized. To address this, I have created different levels of elimination that can be followed at the user's pace and discretion. According to the pharmodynamic model, it can take up to 120 days to eliminate certain IgG/IgM antibodies out of your circulation.[39] If you apply this to antibodies formed from food intolerances, the elimination may be needed for several months before reintroducing them back into your diet. Some people may only need a 30-day elimination to heal the gap junctions and mucous layer of the gut. Once the gut is healed up and the immune system is modulated, you can begin to reintroduce foods that once caused inflammation but now may add health benefits and nutrients. This means a cheat meal during the healing phase can set you right back to where you started if you don't wait long enough to reintroduce the food. Eliminating all food groups at the same time can be too stressful on the body and may decrease compliancy in many patients. Furthermore, some may respond resoundingly to the elimination of just a few food groups. In the Kash Code, the lowest hanging food groups that should be eliminated first include: dairy, grains, vegetable oils, processed foods (sugars, additives, trans fats), and alcohol.

Dairy

Around 10,000 B.C., the Neolithic Revolution began the transition of humans from hunter-gatherers into farmers. At that time, selective pressures forced humans into herding/domesticating animals, including cows. Having the ability to digest milk was extremely advantageous because it made up for some of the nutrient deficiencies in grains, like vitamin D, calcium, and fat. Lactose is the main sugar in milk. Only about 1/3 of humans have the ability to produce lactase into adulthood. Lactase is the enzyme that digests lactose.

The gene for producing lactase into adulthood appeared around the same time as the Neolithic Revolution. Certain bacteria colonization in the gut can also aid in breakdown of lactose. Depending on ethnic background, rates of lactose breakdown can rise considerably. Up to 95 percent of Northern European Scandinavians have lactase genes that allow them to produce lactase into adulthood, compared with East Asian populations with less than 1 percent lactase persistence.[40, 41] In those without the ability to break down lactose, the fermentation in the colon may lead to diarrhea, abdominal pain, and gas.

Other common intolerances associated with diary come from the dairy proteins such as casein or whey. In the initial elimination of dairy, you should avoid all dairy products, including milk, butter, cheese, yogurt, cream, whey, and casein.

During the reintroduction phase you can begin with low lactose dairy products such as cheeses, butter, and yogurts. When introducing milk, please note that some individuals do better with raw milk than processed milk. Raw milk contains lactase, which is removed in the pasteurization process. Furthermore, you can try A2 variant milk from specific cow breeds or other mammals that contain a more digestible casein protein.

Grains

The most infamous toxic compound found in grains is gluten. It is a commonly found plant protein in wheat, barley, and rye. Gluten alone is powerful enough to trigger Celiac disease, which effects about 1 percent of the population.[42] Gliadin, a fragment of gluten, has been shown in vitro to stimulate the release of the protein zonulin to increase the permeability in the gap junctions of the gut.[43] Gluten damages the villi of the gut, which decreases nutrient absorption and increases intolerances to other foods. Pain, swelling, gas, and diarrhea are symptoms commonly found with this disease. However, between 30–50 percent of patients with Celiac disease do not have gut symptoms at all: it will come in the form of headaches, skin disorders, arthritis, depression, and other autoimmunities.[44, 45, 46, 47] This can certainly take place with those even without Celiac disease. Similarly to lactose, a certain percent of the population has adaptability to gluten, while some do not. Immune intolerance to grains can be as high as 13 percent of the population.[48] Individuals with nonceliac gluten sensitivity will have less profound and broad inflammatory reactions to the protein, leading many physicians to miss gluten as the culprit to the patients' suffering.

Aside from gluten, people can react to many other proteins in grains. Each one is correlated with different symptoms and autoimmunity throughout the body. It is safe to completely remove all grains from the diet to eliminate the risk of continuing immune reactivity. By way of nutrient value, you won't be missing out. Grains have low nutrient density and very low nutrient bioavailability, especially when compared to meat, fish, vegetables, fruits, and nuts.[49] Grains fall toward the bottom of the scale, and specifically cooked grains have close to the lowest nutrient availability of any food. The health of grains is largely a myth. They contain a toxin called phytic acid, which can also inflame the gut and binds to nutrients like zinc, iron, and calcium, rendering them unabsorbed.[50] This can be extremely problematic to individuals with leaky guts who already are having trouble absorbing nutrients. Individuals with Celiac disease have to be painfully careful of contamination of foods cooked in facilities exposed to gluten. The smallest residue can set off an immune reaction. Something referred to as cross-contamination can also be caused by foods that have a similar molecular structure to gluten which can fire off the anti-gluten/wheat antibodies. These can be found in foods such as dairy products, chocolate, coffee, soy, eggs, corn, yeast, and tapioca.[51] Gluten could also be found in hygiene products such as toothpaste, shampoo, and conditioners.

Reintroduction of grains

White rice is a good first introduction. When compared to other grains, white rice has much lower levels of phytic acid, making it less toxic on the digestive system and more nutrient available, contrary to the popular belief. There are methods to prepare grains in ways that break down the antinutrients and toxins. Removing the bran from nuts and seeds can eliminate most of the phytic acid. These methods of preparation will be explained further in Chapter 4.

Vegetable Oils

Vegetable oils include safflower oil, soybean oil, corn oil, sunflower oil, cottonseed oil, grapeseed, and canola oil. These oils are high in calories and do not provide many micronutrients. Vegetable oils hit the scene after the American Civil War. Cottonseed oil was originally labeled as toxic waste and used as a lubricant for machines, but after discovering it did not kill cattle, big industries began mixing it into butters and lard. Large consumption of the oils took off in the early 1900s, with the creation of soybean oil, which was marketed as a healthier alternative to animal fats. Today, 86 percent of added fat in the American diet comes from vegetable oils. Prior to the invention of isolated vegetable oils, vegetable oil consisted of less than 1 percent of our calories. As of 2010, vegetable oils make up over 30 percent of our calories.[52]

The fats found in vegetable oil fall under the category of polyunsaturated fats. Vegetable oils are actually touted as heart healthy and today are used almost exclusively for cooking in restaurants and houses across America. However, the more recent science shows they might actually be contributor to heart disease.[53]

One of the steps in the creation of the vegetable oil includes pressurizing the seeds at temperatures over 500°F. This oxidizes the fatty acids, turning them into harmful reactive toxins. Each time vegetable oils are reheated, they become more toxic, which is why fried foods are especially harmful.

Vegetable oils are high in linoleic acid, which is an essential omega 6 fatty acid. However, Americans are getting 100 times more of this than they need. In Chapter 1, we learned that omega 6s are used as substrates in the inflammatory cascade. If omega 6 fatty acids are not balanced in a proper ratio with omega 3 fatty acids, chances of chronic disease increase. Our Paleolithic ancestors had a ratio close to 1:1. However, the standard American diet has them between 10:1 and 20:1.[54, 55]

The half-life of polyunsaturated fats in the body is two years.[56] Its deleterious effects can be long lived. When high amounts of omega 6 fatty acids become part of the cell membrane, they can inhibit optimal cellular signaling, driving mitochondrial dysfunction,[57] and contributing to systematic inflammation and endothelial inflammation.[58] Studies have even drawn a direct connection between excess linoleic acid and oxidative stress.[59] Increased levels of oxidative stress lead to worsening symptoms of autoimmune disease.

Vegetable oils are a food product you should never reintroduce in heavy amounts given their negative health effects. With that being said, seeds and nuts have lower level of linoleic acid when found in whole form. Each oil has a different ratio of omega 6: omega 3.

Reintroduction

During reintroduction, use oils that have better omega ratios and avoid high heating of the oils during food preparation. Seek out seed oils that are extra virgin and/or cold pressed.

Best alternatives include: ghee, beef tallow, duck fat, extra virgin cold pressed olive oil, coconut oil, and flax seed oil.

Grass-fed animal fats have better omega ratios than those that have been grain fed. Omega 3s are also significantly more bioavailable from animal sources.[60]

Refined Sugar

The big sugar industry is infamous for paying off scientists in the 1950s to shift the blame of disease onto saturated fats. This swayed public opinion away from the true deadly culprit for decades and still lingers strong today.[61]

In nature, sugar is sparsely found and is limited to in-season fruits or beehives high up in a tree. Northern populations went without sugar for much of the year. Fruits in the world of our ancestors looked nothing like they look today. They consisted mostly of pits and seeds, were smaller, had much less meat, and were more bitter. The large juicy fruits found in supermarkets today are recent crossbreeds. Naturally occurring sugars from fruits and vegetables are generally fine in the absence of blood sugar problems. However, manufactured table sugar and high fructose corn sugar can wreak havoc on our biology. The United States is now leading the world in per-person sugar consumption with over 3 pounds of sugar per week.[62] It is very easy to overconsume sugar in the absence of fibers. Excess sugar can cause immune dysregulation by feeding bad bacteria in the gut,[63] leading to gut inflammation, absorption issues,[64] gum inflammation, tooth decay, as well as brain inflammation.[65]

High fructose corn syrup is unnaturally produced from cornstarch with its chemical makeup scrambled. High fructose corn syrup is uniquely a staple to the United States. Other countries have substitutes for this ingredient. Large doses of fructose have been shown to contribute to leaky gut.[66]

Artificial sweeteners include aspartame, sucralose, acesulfame potassium, neotame, and saccharin. Artificial sweeteners can be thousands of times sweeter than natural forms,[67] which can lead to a lack of satisfaction from regular foods. One animal study found that high doses of artificial sweeteners can cause alterations to the microbiome.[68] In the healing phase, I would eliminate refined sugars and artificial sweeteners.

Artificial Trans Fats

Naturally occurring trans fats can be found in healthy meats, bone marrow, and raw dairy products. The most well-known trans fat is conjugated linoleic acid (CLA). CLA in the context of grass-fed cows has not been shown to be harmful and contains a different chemical structure than industry-produced CLA.[69] However, artificial trans fats have different effects due to a different structure. They increase inflammation, damage the lining of blood vessels, and provide no added benefit to humans.[70]

Artificial trans fats are found in fried foods, cookies, doughnuts, margarine, candies, packaged foods, and crackers. When vegetable oils are cooked at high temperatures, they produce high amounts of harmful trans fats.

Food Additives

Food additives are used with the purpose of coloring, sweetening, preserving, or stabilizing foods. There are over 2,500 legal food additives permitted—none of which existed 10,000 years ago. These additives are also used to acidify, glaze, emulsify, de-foam, anti-cake, and create hyper palatability. There have been epidemiological links drawn between Crohn's disease and the introduction of emulsifiers to a nation's food processing. Emulsifiers may contribute to gut and metabolic disease development through alterations to the gut microbiota, intestinal mucus layer, increased bacterial translocation and associated inflammatory response.[71]

Alcohol

It is no secret that alcohol is inflammatory and can do pretty good damage to the gut and microbiome, as well as systematically.[72] Alcohol is going to contribute to the toxic load on the body, during a time where you need detox resources dished towards reversing autoimmunity. After the initial elimination, you should be extremely cautious with its reintroduction and limit it to 1–2 drinks per week. Alcohol is a very broad category; someone might respond fine to wine but have trouble with the gluten found in beer. Reintroduce one type of alcohol at a time. Ideally, wine should be organic without additives. For hard alcohols, distilled spirits are the cleanest.

In my opinion, transitioning from a standard American diet to paleo will be the toughest lifestyle change you will have to make. However, the paleo diet will put you in the right direction through its proven ability to decrease inflammation.[73] It is important to prep your meals so that convenience does not force you to ruin all your hard work. Eliminating grains, dairy, vegetable oils, refined sugar, and additives will hopefully give you some symptom relief. You may choose to eliminate each of these foods one at a time.

Autoimmune Paleo

Unfortunately, going paleo might not lead to the symptom relief that you desire. There are a lot more foods that can cause an immune response, especially in those with autoimmune disease.

Plants do not have the ability to run away from predators the way that animals do. For hundreds of millions of years, plants have developed defense mechanisms in the form of sharp spines/thorns and/or toxic compounds. Plants don't want you or any other animals eating certain parts of them. Just like any living organism, they want to pass on their genes.

Naturally occurring pesticides in the vast majority of plants in nature will kill you. Plants that aren't fatal are still toxic in moderate loads. This is why herbivores innately rotate their grazing patterns between different plants in order to prevent overloading on one plant toxin. When dietary diversification is disrupted and consumption of a singular plant prevails, the damage causes the population to die off.[74, 75] My grandfather, who grew up on a farm, told me a story of how when the cows consumed too much of a certain plant, he would have to puncture one of their stomachs to allow the toxic gas to diffuse out.

Many herbivores have four stomachs, which allow for an increased ability to break down tough fibers. Our primate cousins have much longer large intestines for fermenting plant fibers into fat for energy. The expensive tissue hypothesis suggests that the high nutrient density in meats allowed our brains to grow rapidly. Because brain tissue proportionally expends orders of magnitude more energy than muscle mass, we had to trade off other energy-demanding parts of our body. So, evolution traded in muscle mass as well as highly metabolic large intestines, which we no longer needed due to the easier digestibility of animal fats and proteins.[76] This tradeoff eliminated our ability to detoxify many of the plant foods of our primate cousins. Different families of vegetables vary in the types of toxins that protect them. Sometimes, plants will hold two compounds, sequestered from each other until chewing causes them to mix together, and then forming the toxic byproduct in the predator's mouth and stomach. Plant pesticides are also known as secondary metabolites, because they don't actually provide any benefit for the plant outside of protection.

Plant toxins in the right amounts can be beneficial to our health. Much like exercise or sauna, acute stress forces our bodies to produce potent endogenous antioxidants like glutathione and superoxide dismutase. However, if you consume too much of a singular plant toxin in one sitting or chronically, it can do serious damage to the system.

Plant secondary metabolites can be broken down into different categories by structural and chemical properties: alkaloids (cocaine, caffeine, morphine), glycosides (cyanides, saponins, goitrogens, tannins, oxalates), proteins (lectins, ricin, antivitamin compounds), enzyme inhibitors, and phytohormones.[77] There is research that both shows beneficial effects as well as increased oxidative stress from plant toxins. As always, the poison is in the dosage. The difference between medicinal and poisonous can be a very fine line. Individuals with autoimmune disease and leaky gut will have much lower thresholds for plant defense toxins.

Many plant compounds have profound pharmaceutical effects, including antibacterial, birth control, or pain killers. But much like modern day pharmaceutical agents, when you alter one pathway in the body, it affects other pathways and can initiate side effects. Biochemical individuality also plays a role in one's ability to detoxify the plant toxin. Phenolics and lectins have actually been studied as potential adjuncts in vaccines for their ability to provoke an immune response.[78] While there are tens of thousands of plant defense toxins, if we focus on the ones found most often in the human diet, we'll learn that the autoimmune paleo diet includes the removal of nightshade vegetables, eggs, soy, legumes, nuts, and seeds.

Nightshade Vegetables

Nightshades are a class of vegetables that are very high in toxins: lectins, alkaloids, and saponins.

Alkaloids bind to cholesterol on the cell membrane, disrupting the structure of the cell. They also act as a neurotoxin by blocking enzymatic activity, thereby contributing to neurologic symptoms like confusion, incoherence, dizziness, hallucinations, and insomnia. Lectin awareness was popularized by Dr. Steven Gundry in his book *The Plant Paradox*. A case study he published on a low lectin diet revealed that the majority of his patients on a low lectin diet went into remission and off of immunosuppressants. Those who did not go into remission had a decrease in inflammatory markers.[79]

Nightshade vegetables

White potatoes	Cayenne pepper
Tomatoes	Paprika
Eggplant	Goji berries
Bell peppers	

There are many different types of lectins, gluten being the most infamous. Lectins stimulate inflammatory immune reactions in the body and the proliferation of T cells.[80, 81] One type of lectin called ricin has been used in assassinations and was the silent killer of choice by Heisenberg in the TV series *Breaking Bad*. The ricin consumed by eating 5 raw castor beans can be fatal. Another lectin found in beans, phytohemagglutinin (PHA), can have crippling effects in the gut. PHA bind directly to gut wall cells, damaging them and allowing for bacteria to translocate across the protective mucus barrier, thereby causing an immune reaction.[82, 83]

Soy

The majority of soy products in the United States are GMO (genetically modified organisms) or grown with pesticides.[84] Soy contains phytic acid and phytoestrogens. Evidence is mixed whether plant estrogens significantly alter hormones in the body. If soy is the main source of protein in the diet, it can be problematic. Soy intolerance alone can cause immune problems.

Best way to reintroduce: Choose non-GMO fermented soy.

Eggs

Eggs are a common intolerance due to a cross-reaction with gluten antibodies. Also, a structure called lysozyme in the egg white can be reactive. Other times individuals may not do as well with the egg yolk.

Reintroduction: Go with pasture raised eggs, which are higher in nutrient density. Initially, begin with the egg yolk, and then eventually move on to the whole egg.

Legumes, Nuts, and Seeds

Beans, beans, they're good for your heart
The more you eat them, the more you fart,
The more you fart the better you feel
So eat your beans with every meal.

As per the children's rhyme, beans can cause tremendous gastric distress. They are chock-full of phytic acid, lectins, and enzyme inhibitors. Legumes are typically excluded from the regular paleo diet. However, given the huge adjustment of initially eliminating all processed foods, grains, and diary, I have selected for legumes to be eliminated in the next tier. Nuts and seeds are similar to legumes in terms of antinutrient composition. The seed of a plant contains the DNA for future offspring; therefore, plants have a serious interest in protecting their seed, which is why it is the most toxic part of the plant.

Enzyme inhibitors can prevent the digestion of food, contributing to SIBO. Many of us will be sad to realize that coffee comes from a seed. Coffee can be problematic for several reasons, including its cross reactivity with gluten and the acrylamides produced as a result from the high-temperature roasting of the beans. Acrylamides are classified as a carcinogen.[85] Furthermore, nuts, seeds, and legumes have high omega 6 content and can contribute to inflammation.

Omega 6 and Omega 3 in seeds [86]

Food	Omega 6 (mg per 100g)	Omega 3	Ratio
Almonds	12065	6	2010.8 : 1
Sunflower seeds	23048	74	311.5 : 1
Cashews	7782	62	125.5 : 1
Pumpkin seeds	8759	77	113.8 : 1
Hazelnut	7832	87	90 : 1
Pistachios	13200	254	51 : 1
Chia seeds	5785	17552	1 : 3

Low FODMAP

An alternative approach to the autoimmune paleo diet is the low FODMAP diet.

FODMAPs are a class of short chain carbohydrates that are digested by bacteria. They can lead to an overgrowth of bacteria in the small intestines. FODMAP stands for: fermented oligosaccharides, disaccharides, monosaccharides, and polyols. The Low FODMAP diet has been shown to decrease gut symptoms of pain, bloating, constipation, diarrhea, distention, and gas. By limiting FODMAPs, the overgrowth of bad bacteria improves.[87]

Foods to eliminate on a low-FODMAP diet

Fruits	Apple, mango, pear, watermelon, fruit juices, fructose sweeteners, honey, apricot, prune, avocado, cherry, lychee, plum, blackberry
Dairy	Milk, soft cheeses, creams
Vegetables	Artichokes, asparagus, broccoli, beets, cabbage, Brussels sprouts, garlic, onions, shallot, leek, eggplant, fennel, okra, cauliflower, corn, mushroom, green bell pepper
Grains	Wheat and rye
Nuts/seeds/legumes	Pistachio, chickpeas, kidney beans, soybeans, lentils
Fibers/herbs/sweeteners	Chicory, inulin, dandelion, xylitol, maltitol, sorbitol, mannitol, isomalt

Foods allowed on low-FODMAP diet

Fruits	Banana, blueberry, grapefruit, lime, raspberry, strawberry, cantaloupe, grape, lemon, passion fruit, orange, kiwi, honeydew, cranberry
Dairy	Lactose-free milk, rice milk, hard cheeses, lactose free yogurts
Vegetable	Bok choy, pumpkin, zucchini, yam, squash, potato, bean shoots, parsnip, spinach, turnip, tomato, red bell pepper, sweet potato, green beans, lettuce carrot, olives, celery, bamboo shoots, alfalfa
Grains	Gluten-free, oats, psyllium, quinoa, millet

Fibers/herbs/ sweeteners	Basil, ginger, mint, thyme, rosemary, oregano, parsley, chili, coriander, sucrose sugar, molasses

Carnivore Diet

After trying the autoimmune paleo or low-FODMAP diet, some individuals like myself will STILL not see the relief that they desperately need. Unidentified food triggers still exist in the diet. Now that you are aware of plant toxins, the next step would be to eliminate all plant foods and consume exclusively animal products. This is commonly referred to as the carnivore diet.

The very restrictive carnivore diet is for individuals who have severe immune responses to plant toxins across the board. On average, people eat 1.5g of natural plant pesticides a day.[88] Those who consume an above average servings of plants will consume much higher amounts. 99.9 percent of plant pesticide consumption comes from the natural form in plants, not artificial. Micrograms of plant-derived pharmaceutical drugs have the ability to alter our biochemistry. For those who are sensitive to plants, slight consumption can trigger a response. We want to do our best to minimize plants toxins during this elimination as much as possible.

For early humans, our ability to taste bitter substances would have prevented foragers from consuming many of the bitter compounds found in nature. Innovation, a double-edged sword, has fortified bitter substances with sweet compounds making them palatable. This overrides some of our built-in mechanisms such as palate fatigue or sensory-specific satiety to prevent us from overconsuming the same plant. Taste receptor sites on the cilia of the lung are similar to those on the tongue, and bitter substances cause the cilia to increase motility to remove the substances from the airways.[89]

Wheat, rice, and corn make up the majority of the plant food consumption in the world. Compare this to the hunter-gatherers of the Tlokwa tribe of Botswana, who consume 126 different plant species.[90] Some of these tribes reserve certain plants exclusively for famines. The toxic load of overconsuming the same plant can catch up to us.

Certain individuals may be reluctant to try such a restrictive carnivore diet to heal their gut because they are worried about nutrient deficiencies. However, micronutrients are much more bioavailable from animal foods than plant foods. Micronutrients from plant foods must be converted into usable forms in our bodies compared to the already usable forms from animal sources. Therefore, plant micronutrients are converted into usable forms through biochemical pathways in the body, which end up with a much smaller yield of nutrients. Vitamin D3, vitamin A (retinol), DHA, and vitamin K2, are some examples of nutrients in animals that can be used readily. In plants, these nutrients appear as vitamin D2, Beta-carotene, ALA, or vitamin K1. They must undergo structural changes in the body whereby much of these nutrients are lost in the process. Unfortunately, antinutrients in plants can also bind to the nutrients and render them useless as they are escorted into the stools and excretions of the body. In order to get all the nutrients necessary, it is important to consume the animal "nose to tail," meaning the organ meats as well. Often overlooked, organ meats are the most nutrient-dense foods found in nature. According to the Lalonde scale they are 18 times more nutrient dense than grains and 11 times more nutrient dense than cooked vegetables.[91] Interestingly, the first things animals and hunter-gatherers consume after a kill are the organ meats! Liver is the most prized organ. If organ meats are not palatable to you, you can consume them in desiccated pill form.

Humans can get ample amounts of all the necessary micronutrients from animals. Some interventional trials show that increased fruit/vegetable intake either has no antioxidant effect or actually increases markers of oxidative stress.[92, 93, 94] These trials show a differing perspective from the research that shows the benefits of plant foods. The health benefits derived from plants is highly contextual. In the *Carnivore Code*, Dr. Paul Saladino takes a deep dive into debunking the myth that meat is bad for humans from a cholesterol, cancer, and longevity perspective. It is very important that the meat is from a quality source. Factory farming produces suboptimal meat full of contaminants including antibiotics, vaccines, unnaturally fed diet, overcrowding, as well as various other stressors. The better alternative is grass-fed, grass-finished, and pasture-raised meat. Grass-fed animals consume foods that are evolutionally consistent with their bodies, thus lead to more nutrient density and better omega ratios. Pasture-raised refers to the ability of animals to roam about freely with the absence of overcrowding.

When it's time to reintroduce plant foods, you may want to prepare plant foods in a way that breaks down the plant toxins. Indigenous peoples have been using plant detoxifying methods for tens for thousands of years. It can be done through fermenting, soaking, sprouting, or roasting. These processes break down the harmful compounds found in plants and make them more digestible.

Isothiocyanates

Isothiocyanate is a toxin produced in Brassica vegetables; it is a sulfur-producing toxin. For those unable to properly detox, this toxin may produce a hefty amount of smelly farts. The most well-studied isothiocyanate is sulforaphane, which is found in broccoli seeds. Sulforaphane is only created when chewed because the substrates to create the toxin are held in different compartments of the cell. Although some researchers will refer to sulforaphane as an antioxidant, many others refer to it as the opposite because it has been shown to increase oxidative stress and free radicals in human cell cultures.[95, 96, 97] Isothiocyanates have also been nicknamed goitrogens for their proclivity for causing thyroid damage and autoimmunity.[98, 99, 100] There are acute health benefits related to this the toxin, but it should be avoided for those suffering autoimmunity, especially if it is thyroid-related. Popular juicing of high dosages of brassica vegetables can be very dangerous.

Brassica Vegetables

Broccoli	Cauliflower	Watercress
Cabbage	Brussels Sprouts	Mustard
Collard Greens	Kale	Turnip
Cabbage	Bok Choy	

Oxalate Intolerance

Oxalates are a waste product produced by the metabolism of protein in our body and are excreted accordingly. Plants can be very high in oxalates. In fact, when oxalates form with calcium, they become the number one cause of kidney stones. In high amounts, oxalates can cause kidney damage.[101] In rare cases, individuals unable to detoxify oxalates have been killed by 3,500 mg consumed in one day, which is attainable in juice cleanses.[102, 103] Autopsy studies have shown that individuals with thyroid autoimmunity have higher levels of oxalate deposition throughout the body.[104]

Foods high in oxalates

Turmeric powder	Potatoes	Black Pepper
Spinach	Beets	Grains
Almond	Kale	Beans
Miso soup	Chocolate	

Salicylates

Salicylates are a plant toxin known to disrupt hormones in the body. They can cause hypersensitivities and are associated with headaches, asthma, rashes, and tinnitus. A low-salicylate diet has been shown to improve respiratory symptoms.[105]

Foods high in salicylates

Asparagus	Blackberries
Almonds	Coconuts / Coconut oil
Avocados	Tomatoes
Cherries	Eggplant

Fish / Seafood

Fish are a good source of omega 3 fatty acids, fat-soluble vitamins, and other micronutrients. With fish it is important to navigate toward species that have lower levels of mercury. Always go for wild, but even certain types of wild fish can have appreciable amounts of mercury.

Safest fish/seafood choices

Anchovy	Herring	Cod
Clam	Lobster	Oyster
Crab	Sardines	Scallop
Flounder	Shrimp	

Occasional

Salmon	Tilapia	Snapper
Yellowfin Tuna	Mahi Mahi	

Avoid

King Mackerel	Swordfish	Marlin
Shark	Bigeye/Bluefin Tuna	

Wild Meats

Around the same time as the Neolithic Revolution for farming, humans also began domesticating animals. Initially, domestication bred animals to be docile and dependent versions of their ancestors. With time, manmade evolution stressed the need for production, transportation, and aesthetics. Although breeding was slow and stayed local, this situation changed dramatically about 200 years ago.[106]

The genetic diversity of domesticated animals drastically decreased as humans bred animals for uber-specific characteristics. Mass global domestication and distribution of animals has made it convenient to limit which animals are consumed. As humans, we only consume 0.0002 percent of known land animal species. The bottle necking of a species' genetic variability creates the potential for issues. It's well known that the mating of two beings with closely related genetics creates many health consequences. Inbred animals have increased disease, infection, inflammation, and micronutrient deficiencies. One of the major health consequences associated with domesticated meats is the increase in amyloid proteins. Amyloid proteins are misfolded protein structures in the body that are created from systematic inflammation and lead to disease. When consuming these animals, amyloid structures that are indigestible can accumulate in specific tissue or systemically in humans. Amyloids play a role in humans with autoimmune and degenerative diseases. Research shows that high consumption of amyloids can be transmitted between species and lead to inflammatory diseases/amyloidosis.[107] Of course, healthy pasture-raised animals not exposed to the stressors of factory farming will have fewer amyloid proteins.

Unfortunately, there are still risks for individuals in a delicate autoimmune state, especially when terms like pasture-fed, cage-free, free-range, and grass-finished are poorly enforced. Furthermore, excessive bioaccumulation of toxins in the soil from the past can still be present in farms that are currently "organic" and free of chemicals.

The next step of the elimination diet is switching over to wild meats. Wild meats are more evolutionarily consistent and have not been tampered with at the genetic level, mitigating the production of amyloids.

Wild meats

Bison	Elk	Pheasant
Venison	Boar	Wild turkey
	Quail	

Amines are chemical byproducts of high protein foods. They are broken down by enzymes, including the enzyme monoamine oxidase (MAO). Those who are low in this enzyme may express symptoms of depression, migraines, and headaches. Amines are high in meats that are charred, aged, overcooked, or processed.

Ways to mitigate amines

- Consume fresh meats (without preservatives, additives, or aging)
- Consume fresh fruits (less ripe is better)
- Avoid dried, canned, and preserved fruits

Histamine Intolerance

Histamine is a common amine found in foods that can be inflammatory. An enzyme called diamine oxidase (DAO) normally breaks it down in the digestive tract. Individuals with low levels of DAO (genetic, environmental) may express symptoms of swollen eyes, itchy skin, neurological symptoms, or rashes. As you may remember histamine is active in the inflammatory response of bringing blood to an area to stimulate swelling.

Foods high in histamines include beers, wines, kombucha, fermented foods like sauerkraut, vinegar, kefir, and bone broth (bone stock is a better choice). Meats can have high levels if they are cured or smoked.

You can supplement with desiccated kidney in pill form which contains high levels of the enzyme diamine oxidase.

Sulfur Intolerance

Sulfur is an element needed by the body for many biochemical processes. When the gut is out of homeostasis, it can cause a disruption in the breakdown and utilization of sulfur, thus leading to symptoms that contribute to further disruption of gut health. Individuals with a sulfur intolerance need to go more plant-based until sulfur-reducing bacteria rebalance and the gut epithelium has been healed. Amino acids methionine and cysteine contain high levels of sulfur. High levels of saturated fat also feed sulfur-reducing bacteria.

If there is no histamine or sulfur intolerance, slow cooking meat in a crock pot can break down the proteins rendering them much easier to digest. This can really help someone who's struggling with the breakdown and digestion of meats.

For histamine or sulfur intolerance AVOID

Dried Fruit	Allium Vegetables: onions, garlic, chives, leeks, shallots
Bone Broth	
Arugula	Papaya/Pineapple
Soybeans	Red Meat
Asparagus	Coconut oil
Almonds and Brazil Nuts	Eggs
Brassica vegetables	Chocolate
Grains	Pork

For histamine or sulfur intolerance CONSUME

Beans/lentils/legumes (if tolerated)	Beets
Fresh fruit	Squash/potatoes/yams/pumpkin
Carrots	Artichokes
Nuts/Seeds	Rice
Mushrooms	Fatty Fish
Zucchini	Dark Poultry
Corn	Avocados

Slowly reintroduce foods that are high in sulfur and see how you tolerate them.

When humans consume foods that we were not evolved to tolerate, an increase in oxidative stress will occur and lead to a cascade of immune dysregulation. We may even have to adopt a diet that is not optimal for the long term in order to heal the gut. After you are able to identify the food triggers in your diet, you can begin to reintroduce foods. To begin with, I recommend reintroducing only one food item per week. As this is quite a rigorous process, I recommend working with a functional medicine physician along the way to ensure your safety.

NOTES

1   Iorgulescu, G. (2009). *Saliva between normal and pathological. important factors in determining systemic and oral health*. Journal of medicine and life. Retrieved from https://www.ncbi.nlm.nih.gov/pmc/articles/PMC5052503.

2   McLauchlan, G.; Fullarton, G. M.; Crean, G. P.; McColl, K. E. "Comparison of Gastrin Body and Antral pH: A 24 Hour Ambulatory Study in Healthy Volunteers," Gut 30, no.5 (1989): 573–8.

3   Helander, H. F. and Fändriks, L. (2014a). Surface area of the digestive tract – revisited. *Scandinavian Journal of Gastroenterology, 49*(6), 681–689. https://doi.org/10.3109/00365521.2014.898326.

4   *Gastrointestinal transit: How long does it take?* Retrieved from http://www.vivo.colostate.edu/hbooks/pathphys/digestion/basics/transit.html.

5   Baid, H. *A Critical Review of Auscultating Bowel Sounds*. Research Gate. Retrieved from https://www.researchgate.net/publication/40453686_A_ critical_review_of_auscultating_bowel_sounds.

6   Vighi, G.; Marcucci, F.; Sensi, L.; Di Cara, G.; Frati, F. (2008). Allergy and the gastrointestinal system. *Clinical and Experimental Immunology*, *153*(Suppl 1), 3–6. https://doi.org/10.1111/j.1365-2249.2008.03713.x.

7   Mu, Q.; Kirby, J.; Reilly, C. M.; Luo, X. M. (2017). Leaky gut as a danger signal for autoimmune diseases. *Frontiers in Immunology*, *8*, 598. https:// doi.org/10.3389/fimmu.2017.00598.

8   Cell Press. (2016, May 11). *What's LPS Got to Do With It?* Cell Host and Microbe. Retrieved from https://cpb-us-w2.wpmucdn.com/voices. uchicago.edu/dist/e/1480/files/2019/07/Whats-LPS-got-to-do-with-it.pdf.

9   Salama, S. M.; Gwaram, N. S.; AlRashdi, A. S.; Khalifa, S. A. M.; Abdulla, M. A.; Ali, H. M.; El-Seedi, H. R. (2016). A zinc morpholine complex prevents hcl/ethanol-induced gastric ulcers in a rat model. *Scientific Reports*, *6*, 29646. https://doi.org/10.1038/srep29646.

10   Levin, L. G.; Mal'tsev, G. I.; Gapparov, M. M. (1978). [Effect of thiamine deficiency in hydrochloric acid secretion in the stomach]. *Voprosy Pitaniia*, *5*, 36–40.

11   Quigley, E. M. M. (2019). The spectrum of small intestinal bacterial overgrowth(Sibo). *Current Gastroenterology Reports*, *21*(1), 3. https://doi. org/10.1007/s11894-019-0671-z.

12   Pandol, S. J. (2010). *Regulation of whole-organ pancreatic secretion*. Morgan & Claypool Life Sciences. https://www.ncbi.nlm.nih.gov/books/ NBK54132.

13   Esplugues, J. V.; Barrachina, M. D.; Beltrán, B.; Calatayud, S.; Whittle, B. J.; Moncada, S. (1996, Dec. 10). *Inhibition of gastric acid secretion by stress: A protective reflex mediated by cerebral nitric oxide*. Proceedings of the National Academy of Sciences of the United States of America. Retrieved from https://www.ncbi.nlm.nih.gov/pmc/articles/PMC26223.

14   Murphy, G. M. (1998, Feb. 1). *Depressing acid, deconjugating bile*. Gut. Retrieved from https://gut.bmj.com/content/42/2/154.

15   Howard, G. and Wo, J. *Fat soluble Vitamin, B12 and iron deficiency in patients WITH COLIFORM SMALL Intestinal bacterial Overgrowth (SIBO)*. Proceedings of IMPRS. Retrieved from https://journals.iupui.edu/ index.php/IMPRS/article/view/22706.

16   Center, L. U. M. *Evaluation of rate of depression and anxiety In Patients... : Official Journal of the American College OF Gastroenterology: Acg*. LWW. Retrieved from https://journals.lww.com/ajg/Fulltext/2017/10001/ Evaluation_of_Rate_of_Depression_and_Anxiety_in.451.aspx.

17   *Gut health and autoimmune disease - research suggests digestive abnormalities may be the underlying cause*. Today's Dietitian. Retrieved from https://www.todaysdietitian.com/newarchives/021313p38.shtml.

18   Pimentel, M.; Wallace, D.; Hallegua, D.; Chow, E.; Kong, Y.; Park, S.; Lin, H. C. *A link between irritable bowel syndrome and fibromyalgia may be*

related to findings on lactulose breath testing. Annals of the rheumatic diseases. Retrieved from https://pubmed.ncbi.nlm.nih.gov/15020342.

19 Pimentel, M.; Morales, W.; Pokkunuri, V.; Brikos, C.; Kim, S. M.; Kim, S. E.; Triantafyllou, K; Weitsman, S.; Marsh, Z.; Marsh, E.; Chua, K. S.; Srinivasan, S.; Barlow, G. M.; Chang, C. (n.d.). *Autoimmunity links vinculin to the pathophysiology of chronic FUNCTIONAL BOWEL changes Following Campylobacter JEJUNI infection in a rat model.* Digestive diseases and sciences. Retrieved from https://pubmed.ncbi.nlm. nih.gov/25424202.

20 *Irritable bowel syndrome.* American College of Gastroenterology. (2021, Sept. 21). Retrieved from https://gi.org/topics/irritable-bowel-syndrome.

21 Zhao, Y. and Encinosa, W. (2008, Jan.). *Gastroesophageal Reflux Disease.* HCUP. Retrieved from https://www.hcup-us.ahrq.gov/reports/statbriefs/ sb44.pdf.

22 Małkiewicz, M. A.; Szarmach, A.; Sabisz, A.; Cubała, W. J.; Szurowska, E.; Winklewski, P. J. (2019, Jan. 24). *Blood-brain barrier permeability and physical exercise.* Journal of Neuroinflammation. Retrieved from https:// jneuroinflammation.biomedcentral.com/articles/10.1186/s12974-019- 1403-x.

23 Breit, S.; Kupferberg, A.; Rogler, G.; Hasler, G. (2018, March 13). *Vagus nerve as modulator of The Brain-Gut axis in psychiatric and inflammatory disorders.* Frontiers in psychiatry. Retrieved from https://www.ncbi.nlm. nih.gov/pmc/articles/PMC5859128.

24 Vojdani, A. (2009, May 12). *Detection of Ige, IgG, IgA and IgM antibodies against raw and processed Food antigens.* Nutrition & metabolism. Retrieved from https://www.ncbi.nlm.nih.gov/pmc/articles/PMC2685801.

25 Challa, H. J. (2021, Aug. 1). *Paleolithic diet.* StatPearls [Internet]. Retrieved from https://www.ncbi.nlm.nih.gov/books/NBK482457.

26 Powell, A. (2007, April 19). *Humans hot, sweaty, natural-born runners.* Harvard Gazette. Retrieved from https://news.harvard.edu/gazette/ story/2007/04/humans-hot-sweaty-natural-born-runners.

27 Weiss, E. and Zohary, D. (2011). The Neolithic Southwest Asian founder crops: Their biology and archaeobotany. *Current Anthropology, 52*(S4), S237–S254. https://doi.org/10.1086/658367.

28 Snir, A.; Nadel, D.; Groman-Yaroslavski, I.; Melamed, Y.; Sternberg, M.; Bar-Yosef, O.; Weiss, E. *The origin of cultivation and proto-weeds, long before neolithic farming.* PLOS ONE. Retrieved from https://journals.plos. org/plosone/article?id=10.1371%2Fjournal.pone.0131422.

29 Page, A. E.; Viguier, S.; Dyble, M.; Smith, D.; Chaudhary, N.; Salali, G. D.; Thompson, J.; Vinicius, L.; Mace, R.; Migliano, A. B. (2016, April 26). *Reproductive trade-offs in EXTANT HUNTER-GATHERERS suggest adaptive mechanism for the Neolithic expansion.* Proceedings of the National Academy of Sciences of the United States of America. Retrieved from https://www.ncbi.nlm.nih.gov/pmc/articles/PMC4855554.

30 Alex, B. (2020, April 17). *The human brain has been getting smaller since the stone age.* Discover Magazine. Retrieved from https://www.

discovermagazine.com/planet-earth/the-human-brain-has-been-getting-smaller-since-the-stone-age#.XKwEVqZ7nm0.

31 Latham, K. (2013). *Human Health and the Neolithic Revolution: an Overview of Impacts of the Agricultural Transition on Oral Health, Epidemiology, and the Human Body*. Retrieved from https://digitalcommons.unl.edu/cgi/viewcontent.cgi?article=1186&context=nebanthro.

32 Pontzer, H.; Wood, B. M.; Raichlen, D. A. (2018, Dec. 3). *Hunter-gatherers as models in public health*. Wiley Online Library. Retrieved from https://onlinelibrary.wiley.com/doi/full/10.1111/obr.12785.

33 Price, W. A. (2016). *Nutrition and physical degeneration*. Price-Pottenger.

34 Wagh, K.; Bhatia, A.; Alexe, G.; Reddy, A.; Ravikumar, V.; Seiler, M.; Boemo, M.; Yao, M.; Cronk, L.; Naqvi, A.; Ganesan, S.; Levine, A. J.; Bhanot, G. *Lactase persistence and Lipid PATHWAY selection in the Maasai*. PLOS ONE. Retrieved from https://journals.plos.org/plosone/article?id=10.1371%2Fjournal.pone.0044751.

35 Rampelli, S.; Schnorr, S. L.; Consolandi, C.; Turroni, S.; Severgnini, M.; Peano, C.; Brigidi, P.; Crittenden, A. N.; Henry, A. G.; Candela, M. (2015, May 14). *Metagenome sequencing of the hadza Hunter-gatherer gut microbiota*. Current Biology. Retrieved from https://www.sciencedirect.com/science/article/pii/S0960982215005370.

36 Poudel, A.; Zhou, J. Y.; Story, D.; Li, L. (2018, Sept. 13). *Diabetes and Associated CARDIOVASCULAR complications in AMERICAN Indians/ Alaskan NATIVES: A review of risks and prevention strategies*. Journal of diabetes research. Retrieved from https://www.ncbi.nlm.nih.gov/pmc/articles/PMC6158951.

37 Peschken, C. *Rheumatic diseases in North AMERICA'S indigenous peoples*. Seminars in arthritis and rheumatism. Retrieved from https://pubmed.ncbi.nlm.nih.gov/10406405.

38 Williams, R. J. (1975). *Biochemical individuality*. University of Texas Press.

39 Lobo, E. D.; Hansen, R. J.; Balthasar, J. P. (2004, Aug. 24). *Antibody pharmacokinetics and pharmacodynamics*. Wiley Online Library. Retrieved from https://onlinelibrary.wiley.com/doi/pdf/10.1002/jps.20178.

40 Gerbault, P.; Liebert, A.; Itan, Y.; Powell, A.; Currat, M.; Burger, J.; Swallow, D. M.; Thomas, M. G. (2011, March 27). *Evolution of lactase persistence: An example of human niche construction*. Philosophical transactions of the Royal Society of London. Series B, Biological sciences. Retrieved from https://www.ncbi.nlm.nih.gov/pmc/articles/PMC3048992.

41 Bersaglieri, T.; Sabeti, P. C.; Patterson, N.; Vanderploeg, T.; Schaffner, S. F.; Drake, J. A.; Rhodes, M.; Reich, D. E.; Hirschhorn, J. N. (2004, June). *Genetic signatures of strong recent positive selection at the lactase gene*. American journal of human genetics. Retrieved from https://www.ncbi.nlm.nih.gov/pmc/articles/PMC1182075.

42 Gujral, N.; Freeman, H. J.; Thomson, A. B. R. (2012, Nov. 14). *Celiac disease: Prevalence, diagnosis, pathogenesis and treatment*. World journal

of gastroenterology. Retrieved from https://www.ncbi.nlm.nih.gov/pmc/articles/PMC3496881.

43 Rivabene, R.; Mancini, E.;Vincenzi, M. D. (1999, Jan. 12). *In vitro cytotoxic effect of wheat gliadin-derived peptides on the caco-2 intestinal cell line is associated with intracellular oxidative imbalance: Implications for coeliac disease.* Biochimica et Biophysica Acta (BBA)—Molecular Basis of Disease. Retrieved 2021, from https://www.sciencedirect.com/science/article/pii/S0925443998000957.

44 Hadjivassiliou, M.; Sanders, D. S.; Grünewald, R. A.; Woodroofe, N.; Boscolo, S.; Aeschlimann, D. *Gluten sensitivity: From gut to brain.* The Lancet. Neurology. Retrieved from https://pubmed.ncbi.nlm.nih.gov/20170845.

45 Catassi, C.; Rätsch, I. M.; Fabiani, E.; Ricci, S.; Bordicchia, F.; Pierdomenico, R.; Giorgi, P. L. (2008, Jan. 21). *High prevalence of UNDIAGNOSED Coeliae disease in 5280 Italian STUDENTS screened by antigliadin antibodies.* Wiley Online Library. Retrieved from https://onlinelibrary.wiley.com/doi/abs/10.1111/j.1651-2227.1995.tb13725.x.

46 Humbert, P.; Pelletier, F.; Dreno, B.; Puzenat, E.; Aubin, F. *Gluten intolerance and skin diseases.* European journal of dermatology : EJD. Retrieved from https://pubmed.ncbi.nlm.nih.gov/16436335.

47 Feighery, C. (1999, July 24). *Coeliac disease.* The BMJ. Retrieved from https://www.bmj.com/content/319/7204/236.

48 Molina-Infante, J.; *Systematic review: Noncoeliac gluten sensitivity.* Alimentary pharmacology & therapeutics. Retrieved from https://pubmed.ncbi.nlm.nih.gov/25753138.

49 Maillot, M.; Darmon, N.; Darmon. M.; Lafay, L.; Drewnowski. A.; *Nutrient-dense food groups have high energy costs: An econometric approach to nutrient profiling.* The Journal of nutrition. Retrieved from https://pubmed.ncbi.nlm.nih.gov/17585036.

50 Gupta, R. K.; Gangoliya, S. S.; Singh, N. K. (2015, Feb.). *Reduction of phytic acid and enhancement of bioavailable micronutrients in food grains.* Journal of food science and technology. Retrieved from https://www.ncbi.nlm.nih.gov/pmc/articles/PMC4325021.

51 Vojdani, A. and Tarash, I. (2012, Aug. 22). *Cross-Reaction between Gliadin and Different Food and Tissue Antigens.* Retrieved from https://file.scirp.org/pdf/FNS_2013011516575568.pdf.

52 Knobbe, C. A. and Stojanoska, M. (2017, Oct. 14). *The 'displacing foods of modern commerce' are the primary and proximate cause of age-related macular degeneration: A unifying singular hypothesis.* Medical Hypotheses. Retrieved from https://www.sciencedirect.com/science/article/abs/pii/S0306987717305017.

53 Ramsden, C. E.; Zamora, D.; Majchrzak-Hong, S.; Faurot, K. R.; Broste, S. K.; Frantz, R. P.; Davis J. M.; Ringel, A.; Suchindran, C.M.; Hibbeln, J.R. (n.d.). *Re-evaluation of the traditional diet-heart hypothesis: Analysis of recovered data from Minnesota Coronary Experiment (1968–73).*

BMJ (Clinical research ed.). Retrieved from https://pubmed.ncbi.nlm.nih. gov/27071971.

54 Kones, R.; Howell, S.; Rumana, U. (2017). *N-3 polyunsaturated fatty acids and cardiovascular disease: Principles, practices, pitfalls, and promises - a contemporary review.* Medical principles and practice : international journal of the Kuwait University, Health Science Centre. Retrieved from https://www.ncbi.nlm.nih.gov/pmc/articles/PMC5848472.

55 DiNicolantonio, J. J. and O'Keefe, J. H. (2018, Oct. 1). *Omega-6 vegetable oils as a driver of coronary heart disease: The oxidized linoleic acid hypothesis.* Open Heart. Retrieved from https://openheart.bmj.com/ content/5/2/e000898.

56 Guyenet, S. J. and Carlson, S. E. (2015, November 13). *Increase in adipose tissue linoleic acid of US adults in the last half century.* Advances in nutrition (Bethesda, Md.). Retrieved from https://www.ncbi.nlm.nih.gov/ pmc/articles/PMC4642429.

57 Schönfeld, P. and Wojtczak, L. (2007, May 3). *Fatty acids decrease mitochondrial generation of reactive oxygen species at the reverse electron transport but increase it at the forward transport.* Biochimica et Biophysica Acta (BBA) - Bioenergetics. Retrieved from https://www.sciencedirect.com/ science/article/pii/S000527280700103X.

58 Grenon, S. M.; Aguado-Zuniga, J.; Hatton, J. P.; Owens, C. D.; Conte, M. S.; Hughes-Fulford, M. (2012, Sept.). *Effects of fatty acids on endothelial cells: Inflammation and monocyte adhesion.* The Journal of surgical research. Retrieved from https://www.ncbi.nlm.nih.gov/pmc/articles/ PMC3756552.

59 Turpeinen, A. *A high linoleic acid diet increases oxidative stress in vivo and affects nitric oxide metabolism in humans.* Prostaglandins, leukotrienes, and essential fatty acids. Retrieved from https://pubmed.ncbi.nlm.nih. gov/9844997.

60 Köhler, A.; Heinrich, J.; von Schacky, C. (2017, June 19). *Bioavailability of dietary omega-3 fatty acids added to a variety of sausages in healthy individuals.* Nutrients. Retrieved from https://www.ncbi.nlm.nih.gov/pmc/ articles/PMC5490608.

61 O'Connor, A. (2016, Sept. 12). *How the sugar industry shifted blame to fat.* The New York Times. Retrieved from https://www.nytimes. com/2016/09/13/well/eat/how-the-sugar-industry-shifted-blame-to-fat. html.

62 *How Much Sugar Do You Eat? You May Be Surprised!* DHHS. Retrieved from https://www.dhhs.nh.gov/dphs/nhp/documents/sugar.pdf.

63 Brown, K.; DeCoffe, D.; Molcan, E.; Gibson, D. L. (2012, Aug.). *Diet-induced dysbiosis of the intestinal microbiota and the effects on immunity and disease.* Nutrients. Retrieved from https://www.ncbi.nlm.nih.gov/pmc/ articles/PMC3448089.

64 Spreadbury, I. *Comparison with ancestral diets suggests dense acellular carbohydrates promote an inflammatory microbiota, and may be the primary dietary cause of leptin resistance and obesity.* Diabetes, metabolic

syndrome and obesity: targets and therapy. Retrieved from https://pubmed. ncbi.nlm.nih.gov/22826636.

65   Hsu, T. M.; Konanur, V. R.; Taing, L.; Usui, R.; Kayser, B. D.; Goran, M. I.; Kanoski, S. E. (n.d.). *Effects of sucrose and high fructose corn syrup consumption on spatial memory function and hippocampal neuroinflammation in adolescent rats.* Hippocampus. Retrieved from https://pubmed.ncbi.nlm.nih.gov/25242636.

66   Lambertz, J.; Weiskirchen, S.; Landert, S.; Weiskirchen, R. (2017, Sept. 19). *Fructose: A dietary sugar in crosstalk with microbiota contributing to the development and progression of non-alcoholic liver disease.* Frontiers in immunology. Retrieved from https://www.ncbi.nlm.nih.gov/pmc/articles/ PMC5609573.

67   Fujimaru, T. *Sensory characteristics and relative sweetness of tagatose and other sweeteners.* Journal of food science. Retrieved from https://pubmed. ncbi.nlm.nih.gov/22908895.

68   Wang, Q.-P.; Browman, D.; Herzog, H.; Neely, G. G. (2018, July 5). *Non-nutritive sweeteners possess a bacteriostatic effect and alter gut microbiota in mice.* PloS one. Retrieved from https://www.ncbi.nlm.nih.gov/pmc/ articles/PMC6033410.

69   Gebauer, S. K.; Chardigny, J.-M.; Jakobsen, M. U.; Lamarche, B.; Lock, A. L.; Proctor, S. D.; Baer, D. J. (2011, June 28). *Effects of Ruminant trans fatty acids on cardiovascular disease and Cancer: A comprehensive review of Epidemiological, clinical, and Mechanistic Studies.* OUP Academic.   Retrieved   from   https://academic.oup.com/advances/ article/2/4/332/4591508.

70   Iwata, N. G.; Pham, M.; Rizzo, N. O.; Cheng, A. M.; Maloney, E.; Kim, F. (2011). *Trans fatty acids induce vascular inflammation and reduce vascular nitric oxide production in endothelial cells.* PloS one. Retrieved from https://www.ncbi.nlm.nih.gov/pmc/articles/PMC3247279.

71   Partridge, D.; Lloyd, K. A.; Rhodes, J. M.; Walker, A. W.; Johnstone, A. M.; Campbell, B. J. (2019, Dec.). *Food Additives: Assessing the impact of exposure to Permitted EMULSIFIERS on bowel and metabolic health - introducing THE fadiets study.* Nutrition bulletin. Retrieved from https:// www.ncbi.nlm.nih.gov/pmc/articles/PMC6899614.

72   Bishehsari, F.; Magno, E.; Swanson, G.; Desai, V.; Voigt, R. M.; Forsyth, C. B.; Keshavarzian, A. (2017). *Alcohol and gut-derived inflammation.* Alcohol research : current reviews. Retrieved from https://www.ncbi.nlm. nih.gov/pmc/articles/PMC5513683.

73   Whalen, K. A.; McCullough, M. L.; Flanders, W.D.; Hartman, T. J.; Judd, S; Bostick, R. M. *Paleolithic and mediterranean diet pattern scores are inversely associated with biomarkers of inflammation and oxidative balance in adults.* The Journal of nutrition. Retrieved from https://pubmed. ncbi.nlm.nih.gov/27099230.

74   Freeland, W. J. and Janzen, D. H. (1974, June). *Strategies in Herbivory by Mammals: The Role of Plant Secondary Compounds.* JSTOR. Retrieved from https://www.jstor.org/stable/2459891?seq=1.

75   Molyneux, R. J. (1992). *Plant Toxins and Palatability in Herbivores.* Retrieved from https://pubag.nal.usda.gov/download/22035/PDF.

76   Aiello, L. C. (1997, March 1). *Brains and guts in human evolution: The EXPENSIVE TISSUE HYPOTHESIS.* Brazilian Journal of Genetics. Retrieved from https://www.scielo.br/scielo.php?pid=s0100-84551997000100023&script=sci_arttext.

77   Sekhar, C. and Banji, D. (2011). *Plant toxins-useful and harmful effects.* Hygeia. Retrieved from http://www.hygeiajournal.com/downloads/94900624911.pdf.

78   Reyna-Margarita, H. R.; Irais, C. M.; Mario-Alberto, R. G.; Agustina, R. M.; Luis-Benjamín, S. G.; David, P. E. (n.d.). *Plant phenolics and lectins as Vaccine adjuvants.* Current pharmaceutical biotechnology. Retrieved from https://pubmed.ncbi.nlm.nih.gov/31333121.

79   Gundry, S. R. The International Heart and Lung Institute, & Author Disclosures: S. R. Gundry: H. Other; Modest; GoldenHippo Media Royalties. (2018, June 29). *Abstract p238: REMISSION/CURE of autoimmune diseases by A LECTIN Limite Diet supplemented With Probiotics, PREBIOTICS, and polyphenols.* Circulation. Retrieved from https://www.ahajournals.org/doi/abs/10.1161/circ.137.suppl_1.p238.

80   Pramod, S. N.; Venkatesh, Y. P.; Mahesh, P. A. (2007, June). *Potato lectin activates basophils and mast cells of atopic subjects by its interaction with core chitobiose of cell-bound non-specific immunoglobulin e.* Clinical and experimental immunology. Retrieved from https://www.ncbi.nlm.nih.gov/pmc/articles/PMC1941928.

81   Haas, H.; Falcone, F. H.; Schramm, G.; Haisch, K.; Gibbs, B. F.; Klaucke, J.; Pöppelmann, M.; Becker, W. M.; Gabius, H. J.; Schlaak, M. *Dietary lectins can induce in vitro release of il-4 and il-13 from human basophils.* European journal of immunology. Retrieved from https://pubmed.ncbi.nlm.nih.gov/10092096.

82   Ceri, H. (n.d.). *Lectin ingestion : Changes In Mucin secretion and bacterial adhesion to intestinal tissue.* Methods in molecular medicine. Retrieved from https://pubmed.ncbi.nlm.nih.gov/21374487.

83   Ceri, H.; Falkenberg-Anderson, K.; Fang, R. X.; Costerton, J. W.; Howard, B.; Banwell, J. G. (n.d.). *Bacteria-lectin interactions in phytohemagglutinin-induced bacterial overgrowth of the small intestine.* Canadian journal of microbiology. Retrieved from https://pubmed.ncbi.nlm.nih.gov/3208205.

84   Center for Food Safety and Applied Nutrition. (n.d.). *GMO crops, animal food, and beyond.* U.S. Food and Drug Administration. Retrieved from https://www.fda.gov/food/agricultural-biotechnology/gmo-crops-animal-food-and-beyond.

85   *Acrylamide and cancer risk.* American Cancer Society. (n.d.). Retrieved from https://www.cancer.org/cancer/cancer-causes/acrylamide.html.

86   Wikimedia Foundation. (2021, Sept. 23). *Fatty acid ratio in food.* Wikipedia. Retrieved from https://en.wikipedia.org/wiki/Fatty_acid_ratio_in_food.

87 Nanayakkara, W. S.; Skidmore, P. M.; O'Brien, L.; Wilkinson, T. J.; Gearry, R. B. (2016, June 17). *Efficacy of the low FODMAP diet for treating irritable bowel syndrome: The evidence to date.* Clinical and experimental gastroenterology. Retrieved from https://www.ncbi.nlm.nih.gov/pmc/articles/PMC4918736.

88 Ames, Bruce; Profet, Margie; Swirsky Gold, Lois. (1990, July 19). *Dietary pesticides.* Retrieved from https://www.pnas.org/content/pnas/87/19/7777.full.pdf.

89 Ceri, H. and Banwell, J. G. *Brain evolution, the determinates of food choice, and the omnivore's dilemma.* Critical reviews in food science and nutrition. Retrieved from https://pubmed.ncbi.nlm.nih.gov/24564590.

90 Kresser, C. (2014). *The paleo cure: Eat right for your genes, body type, and personal health needs—prevent and reverse disease, lose weight effortlessly, look and feel better than ever.* Little, Brown and Company

91 AncestryFoundation. (2013, Feb. 9). *Mat Lalonde Nutrient DENSITY: Sticking to the Essentials AHS12.* YouTube. Retrieved from https://www.youtube.com/watch?v=HwbY12qZcF4.

92 Peluso, I.; Raguzzini, A.; Catasta, G.; Cammisotto, V.; Perrone, A.; Tomino, C.; Toti, E.; Serafini, M. (2018, Oct. 8). *Effects of high consumption of vegetables On Clinical, IMMUNOLOGICAL, and Antioxidant markers in subjects at risk of cardiovascular diseases.* Oxidative Medicine and Cellular Longevity. Retrieved from https://www.hindawi.com/journals/omcl/2018/5417165.

93 Møller, P.; Vogel, U.; Pedersen, A.; Dragsted, L. O.; Sandström, B.; Loft, S. (2003, Oct. 1). *No effect of 600 grams fruit and vegetables per day on oxidative dna damage and repair in healthy nonsmokers.* Cancer Epidemiology, Biomarkers & Prevention. Retrieved from https://cebp.aacrjournals.org/content/12/10/1016.long.

94 Young, J. F.; Dragsted, L. O.; Haraldsdóttir, J.; Daneshvar, B.; Kall, M. A.; Loft, S.; Nilsson, L.; Nielsen, S. E.; Mayer, B.; Skibsted, L. H.; Huynh-Ba, T.; Hermetter, A.; Sandström, B. (2007, March 9). *Green tea extract only affects markers of Oxidative STATUS POSTPRANDIALLY: LASTING antioxidant effect Of Flavonoid-free DIET*: British Journal of nutrition.* Cambridge Core. Retrieved from https://www.cambridge.org/core/journals/british-journal-of-nutrition/article/green-tea-extract-only-affects-markers-of-oxidative-status-postprandially-lasting-antioxidant-effect-of-flavonoidfree-diet/D0B0C9719378E7002F87734DA6D91798.

95 Kassie, F.; Parzefall, W.; Musk, S.; Johnson, I.; Lamprecht, G.; Sontag, G.; Knasmüller, S. (n.d.). *Genotoxic effects of CRUDE juices from Brassica vegetables and juices and extracts from PHYTOPHARMACEUTICAL Preparations and spices of cruciferous plants origin in bacterial and mammalian cells.* Chemico-biological interactions. Retrieved from https://pubmed.ncbi.nlm.nih.gov/8827059.

96 Baasanjav-Gerber, C.; Hollnagel, H. M.; Brauchmann, J.; Iori, R.; Glatt, H. *Detection of GENOTOXICANTS In brassicales Using endogenous DNA as a surrogate target and Adducts determined by 32p-postlabelling as an*

experimental end point. Mutagenesis. Retrieved from https://pubmed.ncbi. nlm.nih.gov/21193518.

97 Klause, P. *Health benefits and possible risks of broccoli—an overview.* Food and chemical toxicology : an international journal published for the British Industrial Biological Research Association. Retrieved from https:// pubmed.ncbi.nlm.nih.gov/21906651.

98 Felker, P. and Bunch, R.; *Concentrations of thiocyanate and goitrin in human plasma, their precursor concentrations in brassica vegetables, and associated potential risk for hypothyroidism.* Nutrition reviews. Retrieved from https://pubmed.ncbi.nlm.nih.gov/26946249.

99 Truong, T. *Role of dietary iodine AND cruciferous vegetables in thyroid cancer: A countrywide case-control study in New Caledonia.* Cancer causes & control : CCC. Retrieved from https://pubmed.ncbi.nlm.nih. gov/20361352.

100 Chandra, A. *Catechin induced modulation in the activities of thyroid hormone synthesizing enzymes leading to hypothyroidism.* Molecular and cellular biochemistry. Retrieved from https://pubmed.ncbi.nlm.nih. gov/23117228.

101 Makkapati, S. *"Green smoothie Cleanse" Causing acute Oxalate Nephropathy.* American journal of kidney diseases : the official journal of the National Kidney Foundation. Retrieved from https://pubmed.ncbi.nlm. nih.gov/29203127.

102 *DEATH FROM RHUBARB LEAVES DUE TO OXALIC ACID POISONING.* (1919, Aug. 23). Retrieved from http://www.e-lactancia. org/media/papers/Rhubarb_poisoning-JAMA1919.pdf.

103 *Oxalate toxicosis.* Taylor & Francis. Retrieved from https://www. tandfonline.com/doi/abs/10.3109/15563657208991002.

104 Frishberg, Y. *Hypothyroidism in primary Hyperoxaluria type 1.* The Journal of pediatrics. Retrieved from https://pubmed.ncbi.nlm.nih.gov/10657836.

105 Sommer, D. D.; Hoffbauer, S.; Au, M.; Sowerby, L. J.; Gupta, M. K.; Nayan, S. *Treatment of aspirin exacerbated respiratory disease with a low salicylate diet: A pilot crossover study.* Otolaryngology--head and neck surgery : official journal of American Academy of Otolaryngology-Head and Neck Surgery. Retrieved from https://pubmed.ncbi.nlm.nih. gov/25344589.

106 Teletchea, F. (2019, June 7). *Animal domestication: A brief overview.* IntechOpen. Retrieved from https://www.intechopen.com/books/animal-domestication/animal-domestication-a-brief-overview.

107 T. Murakami, N. I. (n.d.). *Transmission of Systemic AA AMYLOIDOSIS in animals—T. Murakami, N. Ishiguro, K. Higuchi, 2014.* SAGE Journals. Retrieved from https://journals.sagepub.com/doi/full/10 .1177/0300985813511128.

The Microbiome

*T*HERE EXISTS A WORLD WITHIN OUR WORLD, whose inhabitants make up the vast majority of biodiversity on our planet. It's a world which we cannot see, made up of microscopic beings. They exist everywhere: in, on, and floating around us. For millions of years, we evolved to live symbiotically with some, while deploying defenses against others. In this chapter, we will dive into the reasons why bacteria, fungus, viruses, and parasites are pertinent to the prevention and manifestation of autoimmune disease.

Bacteria play a significant role within us: They produce enzymes to metabolize food particles, extract and produce vitamins, and manufacture transmitters. Your microbes also neutralize toxic compounds from food, such as oxalates from nuts and spinach.[1]

Your tiny acquaintances form what's referred to as the "second brain." The species of bacteria living in your gut form parts of your personality, moods, and attitudes via neurotransmitters that include dopamine, adrenaline, histamine, GABA, and hundreds of other signals. They produce the majority of your body's serotonin—a whopping 90 percent![2] Some bacteria can make vitamin K, which is needed for blood clotting, or folate for production of healthy red blood cells.[3] They also play a role in hormone regulation,[4] hunger, and satiation,[5] as well as maintenance of a stable blood pressure.[6] Most important, as described in this chapter, is the role of bacteria in immunity, inflammation, and protection against pathogens.[7]

Bacteria have the power to signal genes on and off inside your body! Your microbiome naturally fluctuates through varied cycles: morning to night, menstrual timing, pregnancy, or by the foods you eat, as well as your life stage. Diverse body patterns have differing needs, thus prompting the gut to facilitate communication around your body. Even within one species of bacteria, there can be stark genetic diversity similar to different dog breeds. Although humans share 99.9 percent of the same DNA, our microbiome can vary 80–90 percent interpersonally.[8]

Humans have more bacteria cells than we do human cells. To promote health, tracking our microbiome should be a pillar of our health, equal to measuring our vitals and sleep. Your microbiome can communicate with your brain through visceral sensations such as a gut feeling, butterflies, or gut-wrenching pain. Collectively, these bacteria weigh over three pounds, the same as your brain! They are thought to be as diverse as over 10,000 species.[9]

Biodiversity of species in an ecosystem is necessary for reliable checks and balances. In one famous example, sea otters are known as an important keystone species along the California coastline. Sea otters eat sea urchins and other invertebrates that graze on giant kelp. Without sea otters, these grazing urchins can destroy kelp forests and subsequently the wide diversity of animals that depend upon kelp habitat for survival. Additionally, kelp forests protect coastlines from storm surges and absorb vast amounts of carbon dioxide from the atmosphere. Sea otter populations directly affect the health of California's coastal waters.

The reason I mention this macro example is because your microbiome ecosystem functions in a similar way. In the gut, you have thousands of species of bacteria in varying numbers. Waste or byproducts from one bacterium is food for another, or can be used to communicate with and nourish cells of the body. The elimination of a microbe or the introduction of a virulent one can destroy the stability of the ecosystem.

The field of research pertaining to the microbiome can be very blurry with many discoveries yet to be uncovered. However, one strong link that correlates with good health outcomes is high alpha diversity. (Alpha diversity is the measure of diversity in a habitat.) High diversity protects all species within the ecosystem because their interactions create stable webs for capturing and circulating resources. Therefore, the absence of one species has a less significant effect. Loss of diversity leads to disease or collapse of the system, especially when keystone species dwindle. In the gut, an altered ecosystem of bacteria is called dysbiosis. In the presence of dysbiosis, once seemingly harmless bacteria can outgrow their niche and cause serious problems to the system. Dysbiosis causes chronic inflammation to the gut wall, which changes the environment to better suit harmful microbes, which then leads to more inflammation in a vicious cycle.[10] Diet, antibiotics, stress, circadian disruption, all contribute to dysbiosis. Dysbiosis has demonstrated its presence in Rheumatoid Arthritis, Type I Diabetes, Multiple Sclerosis, and Autoimmune Liver disease.[11]

The microbes coexisting inside of you are not a random mix of all the species present on Earth. Rather, each species coevolved its own collection of microbes to carry out its metabolic and protective functions. There is a unique microbiome for starfish, elephants, and hummingbirds. There are also specific species and breeds for your tongue, your eye, or your big toe. As a species survives and evolves, so does its biome over the course of millions of years.

In your small intestine, where you digest most of your food, bacteria are present, but in relatively small numbers. Everything that has passed through to the end of your small intestine is on its way out and indigestible by you. Opposingly, the large intestine contains much greater levels of bacteria. Here bacteria aid in breaking down fibers such as those found in an apple, then turning them into food to feed themselves. Their byproducts, especially molecules called short-chain fatty acids (SCFAs), are released, and feed the cells in the wall of your colon (colonocytes).[12] Around 10 percent of the calories present in your food are extracted by the guest bacteria in your colon.[13]

Some bacteria colonies make vitamins live in one niche, whereas others living in another neighborhood may be turning starches into simple sugars. There is competition between the colonies. As in cities, prized parking spaces are competitive real estate. The soft layers of mucus have a limited number of hiding spaces to protect from the harsh rain of stomach acid or bile. Many species of bacteria are hungry for the same nutrients and are equipped with identical enzymes. When the last vestige of digestion exits your body as feces, it's a mixture of bacterial cells, worn-out cells of your intestinal tract, and water that constitute the bulk of your stool.

The Nuances of the Microbiome

Most of us host the infamous E. coli bacteria in our intestine; most strains of E. coli are not harmful. E. coli's waste products turn out to be a good food source for certain bacteria. In this case, the two species will tend to congregate in the same environments, achieving a symbiotic relationship.[14] Although, they can "vibe" for long periods of time in small numbers, they can spontaneously bloom if an opportunity arises and then become an opportunistic infection. There can also be the introduction of a virulent (hostile) strain of E. coli from food or water.

About a year before my Crohn's diagnosis, I had driven to visit my sister, Shantal, who was living in Toronto. On my way back to New York, I stopped at a rest stop on the Canadian side of the border and wolfed down a gyro. It took less than a day to realize that was a big mistake. During the following week, I suffered from stomach-turning pain, nausea, and gas. I had contracted a virulent strain of E. coli. Perhaps, if I had a more robust ecosystem of bacteria in my stomach, the symptoms would have been more manageable. Unfortunately, these virulent infections can cause significant damage to the gut lining.

At first researchers and doctors did not understand the implications of these complex ecosystems and unfortunately in certain cases threw the baby out with the bath water. H. pylori is a bacterium that has evolved with humans for at least the last 100,000 years. H. pylori resides in the human stomach. There was clear evidence that individuals who had this microbe present in their guts had higher rates of developing ulcers, and that the eradication of the microbe resulted in the healing of ulcers.[15] Likewise, it is also correlated with higher rates of stomach cancer and various autoimmune diseases. It wasn't solely the H. pylori that caused the ulceration, but rather the body's inflammatory response to the bacteria that caused the damage.

For decades, doctors fought H. pylori tooth and nail with antibiotics to combat the side effects of the bacterium. Researchers later learned that the absence of H. pylori was linked to an increase in esophageal cancer[16] and increases in certain autoimmune diseases (Lupus, IBD, Celiac disease) and asthma.[17, 18] H. pylori strains vary considerably, yet it's still unknown whether these differences indicate which particular strain will cause disease.

H. pylori is an immune modulator, playing a role in the shifting between Th1 and Th2 dominance. Furthermore, it stimulates T-regulatory cells throughout the body. It also triggers your stomach to increase acid levels, thereby destroying harmful foreign bacteria that may be on your food as well as allowing for efficient digestion before food enters the small intestine. Food that is not properly digested can cause gas and heartburn, which is exactly what is found in subjects who don't have H. pylori.

Why would H. pylori live within us for so long if it did not have a beneficial effect? The majority of people born in the United States in the early 20th century carried the organism. Now, fewer than 6 percent of children born in the 21st century have it. H. pylori is disappearing from humans, most rapidly in developed countries, while it remains ubiquitous in hunter-gatherer tribes.[19]

The major reservoir for H. pylori is the human stomach. We don't find the human strain in other animals. In the context of modern Western lifestyle, H. pylori has side effects that may not have existed in evolutionarily consistent environments. Perhaps if we were exposed to H. pylori as babies, while our immune systems were developing and not later in life, our immune systems would have a healthier relationship with the microbe. In dealing with the side effects of H. pylori, we have created new problems. The following example exposes how primitive our understanding of the microbiome complexities are.

Antibiotics

The antibacterial effects of penicillium (a type of mold) have been put into practice since the times of the Ancient Egyptians, Chinese, and Central American Indians. They all used mold to treat infected wounds. In 1928, a scientist named Alexander Fleming discovered the power of penicillium. He started to discard a culture in a petri dish, but mold spores that had prevented the growth of bacteria around it caught his eye.

Part of the effort during World War II was to scale a cheaper, more potent form of antibiotics for the frontlines. To achieve that end, a collection fund was created for the general public to turn in their moldy foods. A woman was hired to scour the markets, bakeries, and cheese stores of Peoria, Illinois, for samples bearing blue-green mold. She did the job so well they called her Moldy Mary. It was one moldy cantaloupe that changed the course of history. This particular mold had potency orders of magnitude stronger than what was currently available. Plus, when the mold was zapped with x-ray radiation, the resulting mutations increased its potency by 1,000x. All modern strains of penicillin are descendants from that 1943 mold. The miracle of the antibiotic saved countless lives. However, like many good things, it was abused.[20]

Antibiotics are indiscriminate in their offensive to damage all types of bacteria in your body. It can then take months, years, or possibly never for your biome to recover. In 2010, health-care providers prescribed 258 million courses of antibiotics to people in the United States, boiling down to 833 prescriptions for every thousand people across the country. The highest prescription rate was for children under the age of two, at 1,365 courses per 1,000 babies. On average, another 8 courses will be prescribed in the next 8 years. Before the age of 22, children receive about 17 courses of antibiotics. Before the age of 40, Americans average 30 courses of these potent compounds. It makes you wonder what other species besides H. pylori are disappearing from the human microbiome that we will never know about. It's the destruction of the human rainforest from within. There are species we will never discover and never know the role they played. A now extinct species in your gut may have prevented a future lethal pathogen. It takes 1 million individual salmonella bacteria to infect mice with normal microbiomes. However, after a single dose of antibiotics, it only takes 10 organisms to infect them.[21] This convinces me that antibiotics are making our microbiomes less resilient to deal with infections, potentially driving an overactivation of the immune system. Children exposed to 7 or more courses of antibiotics had triple the risk of developing Crohn's disease compared with those who never took the agents.[22] With fewer competitors around, resistant bacteria flourish. A CDC report showed that 30 percent of antibiotics prescribed were inappropriately prescribed.[23]

Another way our bodies get bombarded by antibiotics is by consistent small dosages from animals. Farm animals are fed antibiotics not to treat infections but rather to fatten them up. Yes, that's right, antibiotics have been shown to cause weight gain, a practice used since the 1940s. It is unknown whether this has the same effect in humans.

Subtherapeutic dosages of antibiotics have led to antibiotic resistance of the microbes inhabiting livestock as well as antibiotic residue in our food and water. This does not concern antibiotic-free grass-fed, grass-finished animals, but rather feedlots and henhouses containing tens of thousands of animals. In feedlots, animals are squashed closely together, which allows for rapid transmission of infections. By packing the animals into small, unsanitary spaces, farmers set up the perfect conditions for bacteria to proliferate and spread. The European Union forbade the practice of subtherapeutic dosages to animals in 1999. Since then, the use of all antibiotics in animal feed for growth promotion has been banned in all of Europe.[24]

Antibiotics are found in our water, especially around farm runoff and treated human sewage. Current water purification treatments are excellent for reducing harmful bacteria and viruses, but they do not fully remove antibiotics. A 2009 study of several cities in Michigan and Ohio found antibiotic-resistant bacteria in all source waters, drinking water from treatment plants, and tap water. The amounts were small, with the greatest levels in tap water.[25] Even vegetables have been found to have appreciable amounts of antibiotics as they can be absorbed from fertilizers and feces from animals tainted with antibiotics.[26]

The point is, the total of all these insults to your microbiome can sway you away from homeostasis. There are cases where antibiotics are successfully administered to treat autoimmune disease. They can eradicate an overgrowth of bacteria that may be triggering a dysbiosis or heightened immune response. The dysbiosis may have been caused by modern Western lifestyle in the first place; however, the antibiotic treatment may be necessary to move towards the path of healing.

If young mothers have dysbiosis, they will pass this inflammatory condition onto their children. Antibiotic abuse has generational effects. When someone receives an antibiotic to treat an infection, it is absorbed into the gut and enters the bloodstream. From there, it travels to all organs and tissues, including the stomach, lungs, mouth, throat, skin, ears, and, in girls, the vagina. Along the way, antibiotics encounter and destroy bacteria wherever they hang out. All mixed populations of bacteria include both susceptible and resistant bacteria. The antibiotic eliminates susceptible microbes all over the body along with the pathogen that is present usually in one place.

When susceptible species are diminished or killed, populations of resistant bacteria expand.

The fecal sac of the womb is known to be aseptic. But the germ-free baby eventually comes into contact with the lactobacilli-dominated vagina. The vagina covers the newborn's every surface as it passes through. The first fluids the baby sucks on contains the mother's microbes, including some fecal matter. Once born, the baby instinctively reaches his/her mouth toward the mother's nipple and begins to suck. The baby is further exposed to lactobacilli and prebiotics through the first milk. Lactobacilli and other lactic acid–producing bacteria break down lactose, the major sugar in milk, to make energy. The baby's first food is a form of milk called colostrum, which contains protective antibodies. These species are also armed with their own antibiotics that inhibit competing and possibly more dangerous bacteria from colonizing the newborn's gut. When animals lick their babies clean, it transfers their microbes to the next generation. These initial microbes, colonizing the newborn, begin a dynamic process which sets the stage for the development of the immune system and adultlike microbiota down the road. They activate genes in the baby and build niches for future populations of microbes. Their very presence stimulates the gut to help develop immunity.[27]

As explained in Chapter 1, we are born with innate immunity, a collection of: proteins, cells, detergents, and junctions that guard our surfaces based on recognition of structures that are widely shared among classes of microbes. We have a critical period during the development of our adaptive immunity to distinguish self from non-self. Our early-life microbes are the first teachers in this process, instructing the developing immune system about what is dangerous and what is not. As months go by, babies acquire more microbes from eating a more complex diet as well as from the people who surround them: Those born by C-section are seeded with microbes that have no relationship to their mother's vagina or our hundreds of thousands of years of human coevolution. Instead, their microbes resembled the pattern on human skin and organisms floating in the air in the surgery room, including those on the skin of nurses and doctors and bacteria on sheets from the laundry. Cesarean-born infants exhibit a delayed activation of Th1-type immunity, due to their altered colonization. Bacterial colonization is essential to skew the newborn's immune response away from the allergy-favoring Type-2 response towards a Type-1 immune response, which is essential for pathogen elimination.[28] About 40 percent of women in the United States today get antibiotics during traditional delivery, which means some 40 percent of newborn infants are exposed to the drugs just as they are acquiring their microbes. In cases of C-section, this rises to 100 percent.[29] I was, in fact, a C-section baby. My mother tells the story of how she was pushing me in labor for 24 hours when the doctor alerted her that the birth was going to have to be C-section. Cesarean-born children have a 20 percent increased risk of developing Type 1 Diabetes, amongst other autoimmune diseases.[30]

Fungal / Viruses

Fungi are also ubiquitous throughout the microbiome. Fungal overgrowth can result in symptoms throughout the body and lead to yeast infections, dandruff, athletes' foot, or jock itch. Candida are the predominant fungal species capable of colonizing the gut. Candida tends to be more prominent in diets high in carbohydrates and sugar.[31] Candida produces lots of toxic byproducts so if overgrown it can cause serious systematic symptoms. If Candida gets into the blood stream, it can cause a life threatening situation.

Viruses have also coevolved not just with us but into us; viral DNA now consists of 8 percent of our very own DNA.[32] Viruses as we know them today mostly arrived after the Neolithic Revolution. Before this time stamp, humans mostly lived in tribes between 20–150 people.[33] However, they would have probably been part of a larger band or mating network to prevent interbreeding.[34] The genesis of civilization within the last 10,000 years began the development of small settlements that gradually turned into major cities. Prior to this time, hunter-gatherers had frequently switched camps and left behind their feces, which would have been saturated with toxic waste from the body. But with the advent of farming, farmers, on the other hand, lived among their own sewage and provided microbes with a path from one person's body into another's drinking water. On top of being surrounded by feces, disease could now be transmitted via rodents, which were attracted to stored food. Humans also began the practice of herding animals in close quarters. Cities grew beyond small farming villages into millions of human beings living virtually on top of each other.

Viruses like measles closely resemble viruses that may have come from animals. Peasant farmers living with animals could have allowed for the evolution of viruses to eventually hop into humans. Many of the most infamous viruses are relatively young, including smallpox (1600 B.C.), mumps (400 B.C.), leprosy (200 B.C.), polio (1840), or AIDS (1959). The most lethal epidemics within our recent history evolved from animals.

Large populations allow viruses to survive for generations. Certain viruses like measles would likely die out in any human population numbering less than half a million people. In larger populations, the disease can shift from one area to another and persist. Small populations of hunter-gatherers would not sustain epidemics introduced from the outside.[35]

Epidemiology studies link viruses to either triggering or protecting against autoimmune disease, depending on genetic background, host-elicited immune responses, type of virus strain, viral load, or the onset time of infection. Some of the viruses linked to triggering various autoimmune diseases include the Influenza virus, Herpes Simplex virus, Epstein-Barr virus, and Coronavirus.[36]

The Disease of the Absence

Like bacteria, certain parasites have been living and coevolving with humans for hundreds of thousands of years symbiotically. They have been with our species so long that it is possible that our bodies rely on their presence. Most modern-day hunter-gatherers are hosts to a low load of parasites, whereas populations that have gone through "deworming," or the removal of their parasites, see skyrocketing of autoimmune disease within a generation. Farmers and poor communities exposed to raw nature and less clean environments have much lower rates of autoimmunity then their wealthy counterparts living in hygienic spaces within the same society. It is believed that parasites may have played a role in modulating the immune system; however, in their absence the body is looking for something else to mount an attack on. This is the basis of what is known as the hygiene hypothesis.

The Tsimanes, a tribe that lives in the jungles of Bolivia, had 0 cases of asthma and only 15 cases of autoimmune disease after 37,000 examinations. Living in environments that are saturated with microorganisms keeps the immune system primed, and without these archaic inputs the immune symptom falls apart and can mount an attack against itself, harmless environmental particles, or our own commensal gut bacteria.

The low levels of autoimmune disease among farmers can be attributed to growing up on farms, where humans are exposed to much higher and diverse loads of microbes from animals and dirt. This serves as an education for the immune system during a critical malleable period that sets up the framework of immunity for the rest of a person's life. The immune system builds a fine reception of the microbial world.

In the early parts of the 20th century, the majority of Americans still had parasites. In the 1900s, the American government implemented an anti-hookworm effort. During this time, upper-class individuals experienced significantly higher levels or autoimmune diseases than the lower class. The cleaner one's childhood, the greater the chance of developing Crohn's disease or Ulcerative Colitis. The metrics for the study included hot running water and a flushable toilet. Drinking from a well or going to an outhouse had an inverse effect on rates of autoimmunity. As our nation becomes wealthier, autoimmune disease followed in its wake.

Deworming doesn't only present symptoms in humans, but in animals as well. However, in a way, exposure to more microbes is a double-edged sword. It decreases hypersensitivities in the body, but also increases risk of deadly infection. In today's world we can probably create a scenario of obtaining the right amount of exposure to diverse bacteria, while mitigating deadly infections.

Amerindians—Indigenous peoples of the Americas—had levels of IgE antibodies hundreds of times greater than individuals of Western culture, except without any allergies! In Africa, high levels of Rheumatoid Factor, that's high in Lupus and Rheumatoid Arthritis, is simply indicative of malaria presence. It seems that many of the autoimmune markers we have in the West are used to keep parasites at bay in indigenous environments. Take away our symbiotic relationship with the parasites, and the immune system goes after the wrong target.

Malaria had been an endemic on the island of Sardinia for thousands of years. Genes that aided in the resistance to Malaria were passed on. Today, 1 in 430 Sardinians has Multiple Sclerosis; 1 in every 270 Sardinians has Type 1 Diabetes. Only after the eradication of Malaria in the 1950s did autoimmune disease begin to appear. It is then theorized that the Sardinian immune system was highly specialized to deal with the Malaria parasite, and in its absence the system expresses the negative side of the gene with an increase in autoimmune disease. This is similar to how in Africa genes that protected against Malaria end up resulting in high occurrences of Lupus in descendants living in the United States. Parasitic infections don't only modulate the immune system, but they may very well be a keystone species in the gut ecosystem.

Helminthic therapy refers to taking a specific parasite for allergies or autoimmune disease. During the early part of the

21st century, four Helminthic (parasitic worm) species were domesticated and offered commercially so humans could harness the benefits of helminths as a probiotic without the risk of disease. Although there is positive Phase I data for helminths in humans with autoimmune disease, it is not approved by the FDA, so doctors in the United States cannot prescribe them. There are thousands of anecdotal stories of people going into remission; however, there are also many stories of people getting worse. More research needs to be done on which types of parasites are most effective for varying types of autoimmune disease as well as proper dosing. Parasites increase the production of mucus between your gut lining and bacteria. The presence of helminths lightens the load of both Th1 and Th2 cytokines and creates a surge in circulating in IL-10.[37]

Decades ago, if you told someone that in the future people would swallow pills of bacteria for health, they would think you were crazy. I suspect that decades into our future, we might see something very similar with helminths—it may even become common practice along with your other vitamins and minerals. In the early 2000s, you could only get helminth eggs through sketchy sources. However, in today's world more labs are popping up around the world, where high quality safe helminth eggs can be purchased. I can see the opportunity cost: when someone suffers from the debilitating effects of a disease like Crohn's or Multiple Sclerosis with no cure, it is their life and, when all other options have been exhausted, maybe they should have the freedom to make calculated choices with their health. Perhaps this type of option should be included in the Right to Try Act, whereby patients suffering from a life-threatening disease are allowed access to agents not approved by the FDA, but that have positive Phase 1 data. Although there seem to be benefits to specific types of parasites, other parasitic infections can be extremely harmful to humans, including giardia, amoebiasis, and leishmaniasis.

Action Steps

Bad bacteria develop a shield as a way of protecting themselves from cellular defenses. This shield is called a biofilm. An example of biofilm is the slimy plaque that can build up on your teeth. The biofilm helps keep the bacteria or fungus on a surface, isolating itself within a protected community, and blocks away threats. Biofilm communities can leach on minerals in the digestive tract. Inflamed and damaged guts make it easier for these communities to attach to gut wall and thrive. There are natural supplements designed to break the biofilm of many types of organisms. The idea is to take these supplements to create a harsh environment, uninhabitable for these bacteria. Because of the storm that needs to be made, the patient can feel worse before they get better. Furthermore, something called the Jarisch-Herxhiemer reaction takes place when harmful bacteria die and release endotoxins. These endotoxins can initially make symptoms worse. Biofilm disruptors will be effective for the most common infections. However, for more serious infections, pharmaceutical agents may be used. Biofilm disruptors will increase the efficacy of antibiotics and other medications targeting infections. Biofilms have been shown to play a role in IBD[38] and Lupus.[39]

Biofilm disruptors

Nattokinase/ lumbrokinase	Enzymes used to break down biofilm.[40]
N-acetylcysteine (NAC)	An antioxidant shown to be effective against biofilms.[41]
Lauricidin	A natural surfactant found in coconut oil that inhibits the formation of biofilms.[42]
GI synergy	An herbal blend that breaks down biofilm.
Interphase plus	Blend of biofilm enzymes.

There are a number of supplements out there that have a stack of herbs and enzymes that work synergistically to break down biofilms. Some of the most common ones include berberine, artemisinin, citrus seed extract, black walnut hulls, artemisia, echinacea, goldenseal, or oregano oil.

Among the thousands of bacteria species in the gut there are two main groups of bacteria: Anaerobic (without oxygen) and Aerobes (oxygen-breathing). The most abundant subgroup is Obligate Anaerobes called Bacteroides. There is also a subgroup called Facultative Anaerobes which include bacteria like E. coli. When the Obligate Anaerobes are no longer dominating the space is when dysbiosis often occurs, and a person may develop symptoms. Each species produces SCFAs, neurotransmitters, and various other metabolites that communicate with the rest of the body. Dysbiosis results in the interreference of cellular signaling, and inflammation rises precipitously. The colon is mostly an anaerobic environment; however, gut inflammation allows Facultative Anaerobes and Aerobic bacteria to outcompete Obligate Anaerobes. Under homeostatic conditions, colonocytes utilize microbiota-derived butyrate as the energy; during this process oxygen is depleted at the mucosal interface, generating an anaerobic environment in the gut lumen. Dysbiosis leads to low colonization of butyrate-producing bacteria, therefore allowing an oxygenated environment to persist.[43]

Another pattern type of dysbiosis that was discovered relatively recently includes an overgrowth or outcompeting of hydrogen sulfide-producing bacteria. These types of bacteria produce hydrogen sulfide gas as a byproduct. Hydrogen sulfide has its benefits, but in high amounts can be toxic by blocking butyrate metabolism and producing a rotten egg smell.[44] There are binders that can be taken to bind to the sulfur before it can be used to produce hydrogen sulfide or to bind directly to hydrogen sulfide to take it out of the system.

Lab testing can be a great way to get an overview of your microbiome. It can capture dysbiosis, parasites, fungal infections, bacterial infections, macronutrient malabsorption, and inflammatory markers. Testing the microbiome can be very import for finding out which elimination diet/probiotics and supplements may be most effective. Different approaches can be taken depending on the reports.

Probiotics

The term probiotic has been slapped on countless products on shelves everywhere. According to the World Health Organization a probiotic is defined as "live microorganisms which when administered in adequate amounts confer a health benefit on the host."[45] However, the usage of the word probiotics is not strictly regulated within the United States, and supplement probiotics can be long dead while sitting on shelves or not contain what is claimed on the label.

Although probiotics can be used therapeutically, you must vet the product before buying. Our goal is increasing the alpha diversity of our microbiome. With probiotics, the best strategy to try and achieve this is by rotating different brands and strains. Probiotics typically don't take residence in the composition of your microbiota easily because of the tens of trillions of microbes already rooted in your intestinal tract. However, they don't always have to colonize the gut in order to provide health benefits. Instead of colonizing, probiotics can alter the digestive tract in other ways such as by producing metabolites that modulate the activity of the gut microbiota or by stimulating the intestinal epithelium directly. These effects could happen even on short-time scales, ranging from minutes to hours.

Examples of researched probiotics

During World War I, there was an outbreak of dysentery. All but one solider in a German regiment was severely affected. This solider had his stool cultured and was found to have a protective E. coli strain that prevented him from catching the diarrhea. In the laboratory, E. coli was shown to have strong defenses against salmonella. This particular strain is sold today as a probiotic called E. coli Nissle 1917. The reason I share this is not because I think it is the holy grail probiotic, but to illuminate that different strains are protective against different pathogens. E. coli Nissle 1917 has been effective in the maintenance of Ulcerative Colitis remission.[46]

VSL #3 is another probiotic that has a lot of research behind it. For the highest dosage it may require a prescription with up to 900 billion bacteria in a serving. This requires building up to slowly. It has been shown to be effective in Crohn's and Ulcerative Colitis, and in animal models for Type 1 Diabetes.[47, 48]

Soil-Based probiotics: species of bacteria found in the soil. Before industrialization we had a lot of exposure to these microbes from food, water, and exposure. They have been shown to have benefits on leaky gut and inflammation.[49, 50]

There are many other strains/brands that may be beneficial. Some work better for constipation and others for diarrhea. It may be that we have different ideal microbiota states, or fecal types, just like we have different blood types.

Postbiotics

The beneficial excretions of gut bacteria are referred to as postbiotics. They are made in the form of SCFAs. The SCFA with the most significant effect on GI health is butyrate. Butyrate provides 60–70 percent of the energy or food to colon cells. SCFAs control colonic motility, blood flow, and pH.[51, 52, 53]

When colonocytes don't have enough SCFA, they begin to eat your mucosa layer, which is the protective barrier between your gut lining and your microbiome. As mentioned, the lack of butyrate silences signals in the gut and results in disabling of mitochondrial beta-oxidation. This results in the transfer of oxygen into the gut lumen, which changes the environment, allowing Facultative Anaerobes such as E. coli to outcompete. Butyrate has the ability to silence colonic inflammation, tighten the gap junctions in the gut, and promote the manufacturing of T-regulatory cells.[54, 55, 56]

In supraphysiologic amounts and likely altered ratios, SCFAs can have deleterious effects including the opposite effect by increasing leaky gut. Generally, the part of the gut wall, the "crevasse," which is responsible for stem cell production, is blocked from direct contact with butyrate through absorption of butyrate at the top of the crypt. However, in the case of severe inflammation and damage, the crevasse becomes exposed to butyrate and can slow down the production of stem cells needed to heal the gut. In this scenario, it should not be supplemented until inflammation is managed, and the case becomes milder. Prebiotics can also produce butyrate, probably in safer and more slow-release fashion.[57, 58]

Butyrate, specifically, has powerful anti-inflammatory effects beyond the gut, reducing oxidative stress and managing the production of T-regulatory cells. SCFAs can travel through the bloodstream via the portal vein and have systematic effects and receptors on immune cells, nerve cells, thyroid, kidney, pancreas, spleen, liver, and many other places in the body. Topical butyrate has been shown to lessen the reaction of eczema, illuminating the relationship between the gut-skin axis and collagen production.[59, 60] If your microbiome is not producing enough butyrate, initially it can be taken orally (slow release) or via suppository. Fasting and ketosis can increase blood levels of hydroxybutyrate, which can feed the gut lining through the blood. Patients with IBD have lower fecal levels of acetate, propionate, and butyrate, and higher levels of lactic and pyruvic acids than healthy individuals. Individuals with Type 1 Diabetes also have lower levels of butyrate producers, and Rheumatoid Arthritis patients have lower broad-based SCFA producers.[61, 62, 63]

Prebiotics

Prebiotics are known as carbohydrates that resist digestion in the small intestine and selectively feed the good bacteria in the colon. Many times, this comes in the form of soluble fibers that can be isolated to have a stronger effect. Prebiotics can alter population sizes and lead to the production of SCFAs.[64]

Examples of commonly used prebiotics

Psyllium Husk	Citrus pectin
Partially hydrolyzed guar gum	Inulin
Glucomannan	Fructooligosaccharides (FOS)
Acacia	Galactooligocosaccharides

Fermentable Foods

Fermentation is one of the oldest forms of food processing, and likely began accidentally. It occurs when bacteria break down macronutrients into desirable byproducts. Fermentation acts as a method of preservation against pathogenic bacteria. However, it may have become common practice to break down plant anti-nutrients to increase digestability. The day humans accidentally discovered the production of alcohol via fermentation might have earned a coveted spot in human history next to the discovery of fire.

The earliest documented case of fermentation occurred about 9,000 years ago in southern Sweden, when fish were preserved without the use of salt or storage jars. Instead, they were acidified using pine bark, wrapped up with seal fat in seal or wild boar skins, and buried in a pit. The process required a cold climate to help preserve the fish until the fermentation was complete. A similar process is still used to produce the Icelandic delicacy of rotted shark meat.[65]

Some fermented foods include kimchi, kombucha, natto, sourdough bread, sauerkraut, etc. They generally provide a blend and wider spectrum of probiotics, prebiotics, and postbiotics. This would have been nature's way of receiving all the isolated supplements mentioned in this chapter, but together. Fermented foods have been shown to have a positive effect on the microbiome and can decrease markers of inflammation.[66] Raw milk and raw dairy also provide a wide spectrum of bacteria that can be beneficial.[67]

Fecal Matter Transplant

Fecal Microbiota Transplant (FMT) is a procedure whereby a healthy donor's stool is transplanted into the patient's colon. In theory, the patient's gut colonizes with the species from the stool. Rather than supplementing with just a few species from a probiotic, this approach is more dynamic through the introduction of an ecosystem. Although some patients with IBD have experienced remission, some also got worse with this treatment.[68] There is also a case report whereby FMT was used to put a Rheumatoid Arthritis patient into remission.[69]

It is hard to get a superb donor in the Western world, and it's been shown that better alpha diversity from the donor results in a better outcome. There are clinics that have strict criteria for their donors including: having had a vaginal birth, have never taken a round of antibiotics, have a BMI under a maximal amount, follow a specific diet, have no infectious disease, etc. But before this becomes a standard treatment, there are many questions that need to be answered, including dose, frequency of dose, best microbiome types for specific patients, genetics, etc.

There are companies that will even allow people to harvest their own stool into preservation so if they need to take antibiotics in the future, they can partake in a FMT with their own healthy stool. FMT has been shown to decrease the amount of time it takes for the microbiome to get back to normal after a round of antibiotics.[70]

Rapid-fire tips for increasing microbial diversity

- Polyphenols from coffee, tea, and resveratrol[71]

- Researchers recommend washing hands less frequently when you are not around scary diseases

- Get your hands dirty in the dirt

- Own a pet

- Living in a building with central air systems and windows that open—better airflow correlates to a healthier microbiome

The microbiome can be complex, and there is still much to be discovered. Your gut bacteria produce neurotransmitters and chemical signals that control the inflammatory state in your body and subsequently how you feel. One cannot have optimal health without a healthy ecosystem in the gut. By testing the gut microbiome to see where species are overgrown or undergrown, a tailored approach can then be made to nurture a "healthy" microbiome back to homeostasis. The microbiome can make significant changes in days from altering diet/lifestyle. Knowing about the side effects of overusing antibiotics can allow you to make prudent decisions for yourself and loved ones. Probiotics, prebiotics, postbiotics, fermented foods, FMT, and other interventions can be used to help restore normalcy to the dysbiosis in your gut and decrease the inflammation, hypersensitivities, and leaky gut associated with autoimmune disease. For more information on the latest research on the microbiome you can check out Dr. Lucy Mailing's evidence integrative gut health blog.

NOTES

1   Hatch, M. (2017, Jan.). *Gut microbiota and oxalate homeostasis.* Annals of translational medicine. Retrieved from https://www.ncbi.nlm.nih.gov/pmc/articles/PMC5300851.

2   ScienceDaily. (2019, Sept. 6). *Study shows how serotonin and a popular anti-depressant affect the gut's microbiota.* ScienceDaily. Retrieved from https://www.sciencedaily.com/releases/2019/09/190906092809.htm.

3   Das, P.; Babaei, P.; Nielsen, J. (2019, March 12). *Metagenomic analysis of microbe-mediated vitamin metabolism in the human gut microbiome.* BMC Genomics. Retrieved from https://bmcgenomics.biomedcentral.com/articles/10.1186/s12864-019-5591-7.

4   Martin, A. M.; Sun, E. W.; Rogers, G. B.; Keating, D. J. (2019, April 16). *The influence of the gut microbiome on host metabolism through the regulation of gut hormone release.* Frontiers in physiology. Retrieved from https://www.ncbi.nlm.nih.gov/pmc/articles/PMC6477058.

5   SO;, F. *Role of the gut microbiota in host appetite control: Bacterial growth to animal feeding behaviour.* Nature reviews. Endocrinology. Retrieved from https://pubmed.ncbi.nlm.nih.gov/27616451.

6   Al Khodor, S.; Reichert, B.; Shatat, I. F. (2017, June 19). *The microbiome and blood pressure: Can microbes regulate our blood pressure?* Frontiers in pediatrics. Retrieved from https://www.ncbi.nlm.nih.gov/pmc/articles/PMC5474689.

7   Janeway, C. A., & Jr. (1970, Jan. 1). *The mucosal immune system.* Immunobiology: The Immune System in Health and Disease. 5th edition. Retrieved from https://www.ncbi.nlm.nih.gov/books/NBK27169.

8   Ursell, L. K.; Metcalf, J. L.; Parfrey, L. W.; Knight, R. (2012, Aug.). *Defining the human microbiome.* Nutrition reviews. Retrieved from https://www.ncbi.nlm.nih.gov/pmc/articles/PMC3426293.

9   U.S. Department of Health and Human Services. (2015, Aug. 31). *NIH human microbiome project defines normal bacterial makeup of the body.* National Institutes of Health. Retrieved from https://www.nih.gov/news-events/news-releases/nih-human-microbiome-project-defines-normal-bacterial-makeup-body.

10 Zeng, M. Y.; Inohara, N.; Nuñez, G. (2016, Aug. 24). *Mechanisms of inflammation-driven bacterial dysbiosis in the gut.* Nature News. Retrieved from https://www.nature.com/articles/mi201675.

11 Li, B.; Selmi, C.; Tang, R.; Gershwin, M. E.; Ma, X. (2018, April 30). *The microbiome and autoimmunity: A paradigm from the gut–liver axis.* Nature News. Retrieved from https://www.nature.com/articles/cmi20187.

12 Hillman, E. T.; Lu, H.; Yao, T.; Nakatsu, C. H. (2017, Dec. 27). *Microbial Ecology along the gastrointestinal tract.* Microbes and environments. Retrieved from https://www.ncbi.nlm.nih.gov/pmc/articles/PMC5745014.

13 Inman, M. (2011, Dec.). *How bacteria turn fiber into food.* PLoS biology. Retrieved from https://www.ncbi.nlm.nih.gov/pmc/articles/PMC3243711.

14   Smith, N. W.; Shorten, P. R.; Altermann, E.; Roy, N. C.; McNabb, W. C. (1AD, Jan. 1). *The classification and evolution of bacterial cross-feeding.* Frontiers. Retrieved from https://www.frontiersin.org/articles/10.3389/fevo.2019.00153/full.

15   Correa, P. and Piazuelo, M. B. (2012, Jan.). *Evolutionary history of the Helicobacter pylori genome: Implications for gastric carcinogenesis.* Gut and liver. Retrieved from https://www.ncbi.nlm.nih.gov/pmc/articles/PMC3286735.

16   Testerman, T. L. and Morris, J. (2014, Sept. 28). *Beyond the stomach: An updated view of helicobacter pylori pathogenesis, diagnosis, and treatment.* World journal of gastroenterology. Retrieved from https://www.ncbi.nlm.nih.gov/pmc/articles/PMC4177463.

17   Hasni, S. A. (2012, July). *Role of helicobacter pylori infection in autoimmune diseases.* Current opinion in rheumatology. Retrieved from https://www.ncbi.nlm.nih.gov/pmc/articles/PMC3643302.

18   Papamichael, K.; Konstantopoulos, P.; Mantzaris, G. J. (2014, June 7). *Helicobacter pylori infection and inflammatory bowel disease: Is there a link?* World journal of gastroenterology. Retrieved from https://www.ncbi.nlm.nih.gov/pmc/articles/PMC4047323.

19   Bloomberg. Bloomberg.com. Retrieved from https://www.bloomberg.com/opinion/articles/2016-01-07/turns-out-h-pylori-is-an-ancient-bug-and-also-a-feature.

20   Thomas, J. (2020, Jan. 24). *Mouldy Mary and the cantaloupe - mcdreeamie-musings.* mcdreeamie. Retrieved from https://mcdreeamiemusings.com/blog/2019/8/11/1013vvme5498w77bglwoh5ck4exowx.

21   Blaser, M. J. (2014). *Missing microbes: how the overuse of antibiotics is fueling our modern plagues.* First edition. New York: Henry Holt and Company.

22   Prescott, J. (2015, Dec.). *Missing microbes. how the overuse of antibiotics is fueling our modern plagues.* The Canadian Veterinary Journal. Retrieved October 13, 2021, from https://www.ncbi.nlm.nih.gov/pmc/articles/PMC4668822.

23   Centers for Disease Control and Prevention. (2021, Sept. 1). *Measuring outpatient antibiotic prescribing.* Centers for Disease Control and Prevention. Retrieved from https://www.cdc.gov/antibiotic-use/data/outpatient-prescribing/index.html.

24   Martin, M. J.; Thottathil, S. E.; Newman, T. B. (2015, Dec.). *Antibiotics overuse in animal agriculture: A call to action for health care providers.* American journal of public health. Retrieved from https://www.ncbi.nlm.nih.gov/pmc/articles/PMC4638249.

25   Xi, C.; Zhang, Y.; Marrs, C. F.; Ye, W.; Simon, C.; Foxman, B.; Nriagu, J. (2009, Sept.). *Prevalence of antibiotic resistance in drinking water treatment and distribution systems.* Applied and environmental microbiology. Retrieved from https://www.ncbi.nlm.nih.gov/pmc/articles/PMC2737933.

26   Kumar, K.; Gupta, S. C.; Baidoo, S. K.; Chander, Y.; Rosen, C. J.; (n.d.). *Antibiotic uptake by plants from soil fertilized with animal manure.*

Journal of environmental quality. Retrieved, from https://pubmed.ncbi.nlm.nih.gov/16221828.

27 Houghteling, P. D. and Walker, W. A. (2015, March). *Why is initial bacterial colonization of the intestine important to infants' and children's health?* Journal of pediatric gastroenterology and nutrition. Retrieved from https://www.ncbi.nlm.nih.gov/pmc/articles/PMC4340742.

28 Ledger, W. J. and Blaser, M. J. (2013, Nov.). *Are we using too many antibiotics during pregnancy?* BJOG : an international journal of obstetrics and gynaecology. Retrieved from https://www.ncbi.nlm.nih.gov/pmc/articles/PMC4492536.

29 Vehik, K. and Dabelea, D. (2012, Jan. 1). *Why are C-section deliveries linked to childhood type 1 diabetes?* Diabetes. Retrieved from https://diabetes.diabetesjournals.org/content/61/1/36.

30 Wall, R.; Ross, R. P.; Ryan, C. A.; Hussey, S.; Murphy, B.; Fitzgerald, G. F.; Stanton, C. (2009, March 4). *Role of gut microbiota in early infant development.* Clinical medicine. Pediatrics. Retrieved from https://www.ncbi.nlm.nih.gov/pmc/articles/PMC3676293.

31 Hoffmann, C.; Dollive, S.; Grunberg, S.; Chen, J.; Li, H.; Wu, G. D.; Lewis, J. D.; Bushman, F. D. (n.d.). *Archaea and fungi of the human gut microbiome: Correlations with diet and bacterial residents.* PLOS ONE. Retrieved from https://journals.plos.org/plosone/article?id=10.1371%2Fjournal.pone.0066019.

32 ScienceDaily. (2010, Jan. 8). *Evolutionary surprise: Eight percent of human genetic material comes from a virus.* ScienceDaily. Retrieved from https://www.sciencedaily.com/releases/2010/01/100107103621.htm.

33 *Co-evolution of neocortex size . . . —University of Vermont.* (n.d.). Retrieved from https://pdodds.w3.uvm.edu/files/papers/others/1993/dunbar1993a.pdf.

34 *Prehistoric humans formed complex mating networks to avoid inbreeding.* SMU Research. (n.d.). Retrieved from https://blog.smu.edu/research/2017/10/10/prehistoric-humans-formed-complex-mating-networks-avoid-inbreeding.

35 Diamond, J. M. (1999). *Guns, germs, and steel:* The fates of human societies. New York: W.W. Norton & Co.

36 Smatti, M. K.; Cyprian, F. S.; Nasrallah, G. K.; Al Thani, A. A.; Almishal, R. O.; Yassine, H. M. (2019, Aug. 19). *Viruses and autoimmunity: A review on the potential interaction and molecular mechanisms.* Viruses. Retrieved from https://www.ncbi.nlm.nih.gov/pmc/articles/PMC6723519.

37 Velasquez-Manoff, M. (2012). *An epidemic of absence: a new way of understanding allergies and autoimmune diseases.* 1st Scribner's hardcover ed. New York, NY: Charles Scribner's Sons.

38 Swidsinski, A.; Loening-Baucke, V.; Bengmark, S.; Scholze, J.; Doerffel, Y. (n.d.). *Bacterial biofilm suppression with antibiotics for ulcerative and indeterminate colitis: Consequences of aggressive treatment.* Archives of medical research. Retrieved from https://pubmed.ncbi.nlm.nih.gov/18164963.

39   Gallo, P. M.; Rapsinski, G. J.; Wilson, R. P.; Oppong, G. O.; Sriram, U.;
     Goulian, M.; Buttaro, B.; Caricchio, R.; Gallucci, S.; Tükel, Ç. (2015,
     June 16). *Amyloid-DNA composites of bacterial biofilms stimulate
     autoimmunity.* Immunity. Retrieved from https://www.ncbi.nlm.nih.gov/
     pmc/articles/PMC4500125.

40   E;, H. S. O. G. J. P. O. N. (n.d.). *Novel treatment of Staphylococcus
     aureus device-related infections using fibrinolytic agents.* Antimicrobial
     agents and chemotherapy. Retrieved from https://pubmed.ncbi.nlm.nih.
     gov/29203484.

41   JY;, C. Y. S. K. C. M. J. H. L. (n.d.). *Removal and killing of multispecies
     endodontic biofilms by N-Acetylcysteine.* Brazilian journal of microbiology
     : [publication of the Brazilian Society for Microbiology]. Retrieved from
     https://pubmed.ncbi.nlm.nih.gov/28916389.

42   TJ;, H. Y. K. (n.d.). *Inhibitory activity of monoacylglycerols on biofilm
     formation in aeromonas hydrophila, streptococcus mutans, xanthomonas
     oryzae, and Yersinia Enterocolitica.* SpringerPlus. Retrieved from https://
     pubmed.ncbi.nlm.nih.gov/27652099.

43   Litvak, Y.; Byndloss, M. X.; Bäumler, A. J. (2018, Nov. 30). *Colonocyte
     metabolism shapes the gut microbiota.* Science (New York, N.Y.). Retrieved
     from https://www.ncbi.nlm.nih.gov/pmc/articles/PMC6296223.

44   DR;, L. (n.d.). *Hydrogen sulfide signaling in the gastrointestinal tract.*
     Antioxidants & redox signaling. Retrieved from https://pubmed.ncbi.nlm.
     nih.gov/23582008.

45   Mack, D. R. (2005, Nov.). *Probiotics-mixed messages.* Canadian family
     physician Medecin de famille canadien. Retrieved from https://www.ncbi.
     nlm.nih.gov/pmc/articles/PMC1479485.

46   Scaldaferri, F.; Gerardi, V.; Mangiola, F.; Lopetuso, L. R.; Pizzoferrato, M.;
     Petito, V.; Papa, A.; Stojanovic, J.; Poscia, A.; Cammarota, G.; Gasbarrini,
     A. (2016, June 28). *Role and mechanisms of action of escherichia coli
     Nissle 1917 in the maintenance of remission in ulcerative colitis patients:
     An update.* World journal of gastroenterology. Retrieved from https://
     www.ncbi.nlm.nih.gov/pmc/articles/PMC4917610.

47   Fedorak, R. N.; Feagan, B. G.; Hotte, N.; Leddin, D.; Dieleman, L. A.;
     Petrunia, D. M.; Enns, R.; Bitton, A.; Chiba. N.; Paré, P.; Rostom, A.;
     Marshall, J.; Depew, W.; Bernstein, C. N.; Panaccione, R.; Aumais, G.;
     Steinhart, A. H.; Cockeram, A.; Bailey, R. J.; Gionchetti, P.; Wong, C.;
     Madsen, K. (n.d.). *The probiotic VSL#3 has anti-inflammatory effects
     and could reduce endoscopic recurrence after surgery for crohn's disease.*
     Clinical gastroenterology and hepatology : the official clinical practice
     journal of the American Gastroenterological Association. Retrieved, from
     https://pubmed.ncbi.nlm.nih.gov/25460016.

48   Dolpady, J.; Sorini, C.; Di Pietro, C.; Cosorich, I.; Ferrarese, R.; Saita,
     D.; Clementi, M.; Canducci, F.; Falcone, M. (n.d.). *Oral probiotic VSL#3
     prevents autoimmune diabetes by modulating microbiota and promoting
     indoleamine 2,3-dioxygenase-enriched tolerogenic intestinal environment.*
     Journal of diabetes research. Retrieved from https://pubmed.ncbi.nlm.nih.
     gov/26779542.

49 McFarlin, B. K.; Henning, A. L.; Bowman, E. M.;Gary, M. A.; Carbajal, K. M. (n.d.). *Oral spore-based probiotic supplementation was associated with reduced incidence of post-prandial dietary endotoxin, triglycerides, and disease risk biomarkers.* World journal of gastrointestinal pathophysiology. Retrieved from https://pubmed.ncbi.nlm.nih.gov/28868181.

50 Nyangale, E. P.; Farmer, S.; Cash, H. A.; Keller, D.; Chernoff, D.; Gibson, G. R. (n.d.). *Bacillus coagulans GBI-30, 6086 modulates faecalibacterium prausnitzii in older men and women.* The Journal of nutrition. Retrieved, from https://pubmed.ncbi.nlm.nih.gov/25948780.

51 Donohoe, D. R., et al. *The Microbiome and Butyrate Regulate Energy Metabolism and Autophagy in the Mammalian Colon.* Cell Metab. 13, 517–526 (2011).

52 Suzuki, T.; Yoshida, S.; Hara, H. *Physiological concentrations of short-chain fatty acids immediately suppress colonic epithelial permeability.* Br. J. Nutr. 100, 297–305 (2008).

53 Tazoe, H., et al. *Roles of short-chain fatty acids receptors, GPR41 and GPR43 on colonic functions.* J. Physiol. Pharmacol. Off. J. Pol. Physiol. Soc. 59 Suppl 2, 251–262 (2008).

54 Singh, N., et al. *Activation of Gpr109a, receptor for niacin and the commensal metabolite butyrate, suppresses colonic inflammation and carcinogenesis.* Immunity 40, 128–139 (2014).

55 Peng, L.; He, Z.; Chen, W.; Holzman, I. R.; Lin, J. *Effects of butyrate on intestinal barrier function in a Caco-2 cell monolayer model of intestinal barrier.* Pediatr. Res. 61, 37–41 (2007).

56 Säemann, M. D. *Anti-inflammatory effects of sodium butyrate on human monocytes: potent inhibition of IL-12 and up-regulation of IL-10 production.* FASEB J. Off. Publ. Fed. Am. Soc. Exp. Biol. 14, 2380–2382 (2000).

57 Peng, L.; He, Z.; Chen, W.; Holzman, I. R.; Lin, J. *Effects of butyrate on intestinal barrier function in a Caco-2 cell monolayer model of intestinal barrier.* Pediatr. Res. 61, 37–41 (2007).

58 Kaiko, G. E. *The Colonic Crypt Protects Stem Cells from Microbiota-Derived Metabolites.* Cell 165, 1708–1720 (2016).

59 Schwarz, A.; Bruhs, A.; Schwarz, T. *The Short-Chain Fatty Acid Sodium Butyrate Functions as a Regulator of the Skin Immune System.* J. Invest. Dermatol. 137, 855–864 (2017).

60 Karna, E.; Trojan, S.; Pałka, J. A. *The mechanism of butyrate-induced collagen biosynthesis in cultured fibroblasts.* Acta Pol. Pharm. 66, 129–134 (2009).

61 Frank, D. N. *Molecular-phylogenetic characterization of microbial community imbalances in human inflammatory bowel diseases.* Proc. Natl. Acad. Sci. U. S. A. 104, 13780–13785 (2007).

62 Brown, C. T. *Gut Microbiome Metagenomics Analysis Suggests a Functional Model for the Development of Autoimmunity for Type 1 Diabetes.* PLOS ONE 6, e25792 (2011).

63   Vaahtovuo, J.; Munukka, E.; Korkeamäki, M.; Luukkainen, R.; Toivanen, P. *Fecal microbiota in early rheumatoid arthritis*. J. Rheumatol. 35, 1500–1505 (2008).

64   Slavin, J. (2013, April 22). *Fiber and prebiotics: Mechanisms and health benefits*. Nutrients. Retrieved from https://www.ncbi.nlm.nih.gov/pmc/articles/PMC3705355.

65   Boethius, A. (2016, Feb. 6). *Something Rotten in Scandinavia: The world's earliest evidence of fermentation*. Journal of Archaeological Science. Retrieved from https://www.sciencedirect.com/science/article/abs/pii/S0305440316000170.

66   Wastyk, H.; Fragiadakis, G.; Perelman, D. (2021, July 12). *Gut-microbiota-targeted diets modulate human immune status*. Cell. Retrieved from https://www.cell.com/cell/fulltext/S0092-8674(21)00754-6?_returnURL=https://linkinghub.elsevier.com/retrieve/pii/S0092867421007546%3Fshowall%3Dtrue.

67   O'Sullivan, O. and Cotter, P. D. (2017, May 12). *Microbiota of raw milk and raw milk cheeses*. Cheese (Fourth edition). Retrieved from www.sciencedirect.com/science/article/pii/B9780124170124000120.

68   Levy, A. N. and Allegretti, J. R. (2019, March 14). *Insights into the role of fecal microbiota transplantation for the treatment of inflammatory bowel disease*. Therapeutic advances in gastroenterology. Retrieved from www.ncbi.nlm.nih.gov/pmc/articles/PMC6421596.

69   Zeng, J.; Peng, L.; Zheng, W.; Huang, F.; Zhang, N.; Wu, D.; Yang, Y. (2020, Dec. 23). *Fecal microbiota transplantation for rheumatoid arthritis: A case report*. Wiley Online Library. Retrieved from https://onlinelibrary.wiley.com/doi/full/10.1002/ccr3.3677.

70   Suez, J.; Zmora, N.; Zilberman-Schapira, G.; Mor, U.; Dori-Bachash, M.; Bashiardes, S.; Zur, M.; Regev-Lehavi, D.; Brik, R. B.-Z.; Federici, S.; Horn, M.; Cohen, Y.; Moor, A. E.; Zeevi, D.; Korem, T.; Kotler, E.; Harmelin, A.; Itzkovitz, S.; Elinav, E. (2018, Sept. 6). *Post-antibiotic gut mucosal microbiome reconstitution is impaired by probiotics and improved by autologous fmt*. Cell. Retrieved from https://www.sciencedirect.com/science/article/pii/S0092867418311085.

71   Kumar Singh, A.; Cabral, C.; Kumar, R.; Ganguly, R.; Kumar Rana, H.; Gupta, A.; Rosaria Lauro, M.; Carbone, C.; Reis, F.; Pandey, A. K. (2019, Sept. 13). *Beneficial effects of dietary polyphenols on gut microbiota and strategies to improve delivery efficiency*. Nutrients. Retrieved from https://www.ncbi.nlm.nih.gov/pmc/articles/PMC6770155.

CHAPTER 5

Stress

TWENTY THOUSAND YEARS AGO, Colby is building a shelter on the savanna, when he hears ruffles in the bushes. He is alarmed to find out he is being stalked by a lion; his tribesmen react quickly to neutralize the threat with a communicated effort of slings, spears, and arrows. This is an example of how human experience dealt with an acute stressor throughout most of our evolution. However, this stress was short-lived, and then our body would wobble back into homeostasis, relaxing our organs and glands.

In today's world, some individuals never stop running from the lion. They may be chronically sleep deprived, nutrient deprived, and always thinking about dooming work/school deadlines. Stress in its essence is your body's response to demand. Your body has an allostatic load, or a priority list. When there are mental lions consistently throughout your day, the body pools its resources into fight-or-flight mode and immune function/efficiency takes a seat on the bench.

Your body's autonomic nervous system is split up into two divisions: the sympathetic nervous system and the parasympathetic nervous system. Your sympathetic nervous system is the "fight-or-flight" system responsible for keeping you alert under stress and directing blood to your skeletal muscles. Your parasympathetic system stimulates "rest and digest," and is responsible for mellowing you out and redirecting blood and nutrients to other bodily systems such as the stomach and intestines. You need a balance between the two systems. The sympathetic nervous system increases heart rate and blood pressure, opens your lungs, and dilates your pupils. The parasympathetic system decreases heart rate, stimulates digestive enzymes, constricts pupils, and stimulates the sex organs. The overstimulation of our sympathetic nervous system is a cause of stress-related disease, including high blood pressure, digestive problems, chronic headaches, backaches, sleep disorders, arrhythmias, and chronic anxiety.[1]

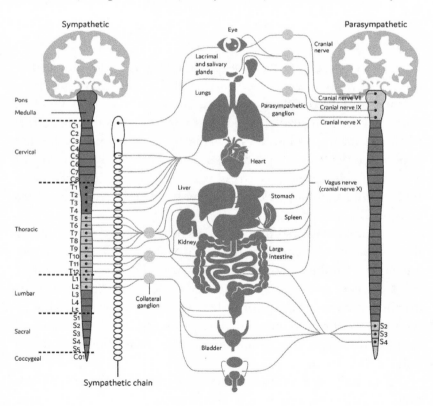

Chronic psychological stress plays an integral role in autoimmune disease and can be a cash cow of tokens into your stress bank that will eventually tip someone into poor health. The same threshold that causes autoimmune disease is not the same level that will put you into remission. You have to go further and beyond to heal yourself and, in this chapter, you will learn about the importance of the mind.

The body is blind to the difference between psychological and physical stress and translates those environmental signals into biochemical messengers. Stress enters the body through our five senses and activates a part of our brainstem called the locus coeruleus.[2]

The body regulates stress through various glands by way of feedback mechanisms. This mechanism is referred to as the hypothalamic-pituitary-adrenal axis or HPA axis. The hypothalamus is located at the base of the brain, and its main role is regulating homeostasis of heart rate, blood pressure, body temperature, hydration, appetite, gland secretion, and sleep cycles.[3] The pituitary gland is the size of a pea and is located at the base of the brain below the hypothalamus.[4] The adrenal glands sit on top of the kidneys.

The locus coeruleus produces norepinephrine (adrenaline) in the brain in response to perceived stress. Once activated, adrenaline-bound neurons send signals to other parts of the brain. Adrenaline carries the stress message by activating the HPA axis and triggers a cascade that produces hormones—including cortisol and DHEA—integral to managing our stress response. The adrenal medulla, the inside of the adrenal gland, produces hormones in response to stress and is stimulated by the sympathetic nervous system fibers, and bypasses the HPA axis, making it a lot faster than cortisol. It is referred to as the sympathoadrenal system, and it releases norepinephrine and epinephrine (adrenaline) for the body.[5] Adrenaline is the booster for acute stress and, in seconds, it can mobilize glucose to the muscles and the brain.

The locus coeruleus plays a role in signaling the corticotropin-releasing hormone (CRH) release from the hypothalamus, which stimulates the anterior pituitary to release adrenocorticotrophic hormone (ACTH), which then goes on to stimulate the adrenal cortex—the outer part of the adrenal gland—to release glucocorticoids mostly in the form of cortisol. Cortisol stimulates the production of glucose, mobilizing of amino acids and breaking down fat, and it has anti-inflammatory effects. The HPA axis works on negative feedback, so as levels of cortisol in the blood elevate, it signals the hypothalamus to slow down its production of CRH.[6]

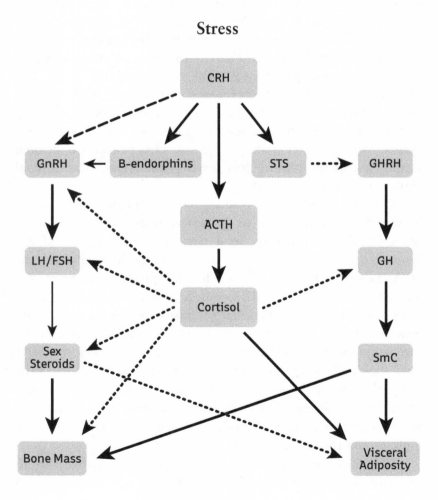

CRH has also been found to be produced outside the brain, in the gut and skin. This may play a role in the gut-brain-skin axis and explain why gut inflammation is correlated with skin and neuroinflammatory disorders.[7]

If cortisol is thought of as a catabolic hormone, meaning it breaks down tissues, the antaganol hormone is DHEA, which is an anabolic hormone (or building up). DHEA is produced in the adrenal cortex and it builds muscle, neurons, and the immune system. It is a precursor to hormones like testosterone. However, chronic stress can cause a scenario whereby cortisol is high, and DHEA is low, putting the body into a long-term catabolic phase, inhibiting the regeneration of tissues including the gut lining![8]

Under normal levels, DHEA strengthens the immune system while also inhibiting inflammatory cytokines, upregulating anti-inflammatory cytokines, and boosting neuro activity. It is low in various inflammatory diseases, but can also be high in the case of obesity.[9] Both cortisol and DHEA and all their sub types need to be at proper levels. There are about 12 different dysfunctional hormonal patterns associated with the adrenal glands, all needing a unique treatment approach, but this is not in the scope of this book.

High cortisol suppresses inflammation/immune function, which might sound like a positive thing for an overactive immune system. However, we do not want a suppressed immune system, we want a properly functioning one. Also, high cortisol causes a shift to a Th2 response rather than general immunosuppression. This leads to a domination of one side of the immune system, which we know spells out autoimmune disease. This immune suppression from high levels of cortisol explains the connection between stress and increased risk of infection. Unnatural levels of cortisol are disrupting the homeostatic balance we need in our immune system to function properly. High levels of cortisol decrease wound healing and downregulate the synthesis of collagen, which is an important component of muscles, tendons, and joints. This is why high-cortisol states are associated with muscle wasting.[10] This is often a side effect of corticosteroid medications. They act to eliminate the inflammation as a short-term fix, but inhibit long-term healing. DHEA seems to stimulate Th1 reactions while inhibiting Th2.[11] This shows the homeostatic balance needed between both cortisol and DHEA and how stimulation of one or the other may modulate the ecosystem to your advantage.

Over time, if perceived stress does not dissipate and the adrenals continue to pump massive amounts of cortisol, the glucocorticoid receptor sites begin to become resistant to cortisol and it no longer has its same effects. This is similar to Type II Diabetes when the body becomes resistant to the signal of insulin after chronically dumping massive amounts of it into the system. Furthermore, much of the cortisol will be converted into cortisone—the less active form of cortisol—and lose the ability to quell inflammation. It is not uncommon for individuals with low free cortisol to have high total cortisol. The body is converting cortisol into the unusable form to prevent the wasting away of tissues. Further side effects of a high cortisol state include decreases in growth hormone, suppression of thyroid function, increase in insulin resistance, and inhibited bone remodeling. This "hypo-cortisol" state is responsible for a boost in proinflammatory cytokines such as tumor necrosis factor and IL-6, and disruption of T-cell signaling. To make up for the lack of cortisol bioavailability and sensitive cortisol receptors, the sympathoadrenal system can be used as a crutch to rev up adrenaline production, thereby producing even more pro-inflammatory cytokines.[12]

Chronic stress causes your body to become less resilient to mitigate the effects of stress load and begin to wear down over time. Overstimulation of the corticoid hormones is directly linked to adverse malleable changes to the brain such as decreasing volume in the amygdala and hippocampus. These are the parts of the brain responsible for emotions and memory. This stress-linked pathway imprints a vicious cycle of constant fight-or-flight mindset.[13]

Adrenal fatigue has become a popularized diagnostic term to describe symptoms of low energy, lethargy, and brain fog. It refers to the long-term consequences of chronic stress eventually burning out the adrenal glands so they stop producing the stress hormones. First cortisol production increases during a period of months to years and DHEA lowers. After this period the body "adapts" and cortisol falls into normal range while DHEA stays low. Finally, in the last stage cortisol also drops because the adrenal glands "burn out" and are not able to keep up with the stress demand. This theory was used as an explanation for the symptoms described above. However, when studied it has been shown that adrenal fatigue is sort of a myth and is often over diagnosed. HPA dysfunction that presents with fatigue symptoms and low cortisol is not caused by burnout of the adrenals in most patients. The problems lie with cortisol receptor sensitivity, the amount of cortisol bound to binding proteins (only free cortisol has signaling ability), downregulation of CRH or ACTH, or infection. HPA axis dysfunction is present in autoimmune diseases across the board for the inability to turn off inflammation: IBD, Fibromyalgia, Rheumatoid Arthritis, Multiple Sclerosis, and other neurological conditions.[14]

In the literature, the rare cases that "adrenal fatigue" occurs and the adrenals are the root cause of the inability to produce cortisol it is referred to as adrenal insufficiency. One example includes Addison's Disease, an autoimmune disease whereby the body attacks the adrenal glands, damaging and inhibiting the ability of the body to produce cortisol, amongst several other hormones. Adrenal insufficiency can also be caused by use of corticosteroids pills, inhalers, or creams.[15]

Another important aspect of the HPA axis is circadian rhythm. Hormones have cycles throughout the day. Disruption to these cycles can cause peaking at the wrong times which will throw off your energy leading to day sleepiness and restlessness at bedtime. There are various hormonal tests that can be used to figure out the patterned dysfunction. However, some tests do not give you the complete picture and can lead to misdiagnosis and mistreatment that can cause further disruption.

Now that we understand the hormonal cascade that takes place, I would like to talk about what gets people stuck in an abnormal stress response. The normal stress response occurs when the body reacts by increasing stress hormones, but over time adapts to the stress (at the same volume and intensity) and decreases the amount of stress hormones released by the same stimulus. There can be a hyper-active stress response, whereby the body continues to react to the same stress by releasing stress hormones at high levels. This can happen in individuals with PTSD, trauma, depression, OCD, hyperthyroidism, burn-out syndrome or other anxiety disorders. Finally, there can be a hypoactive stress response, whereby the body fails to respond to the external stress with ample amounts of stress hormones. A hypoactive response can be seen in Fibromyalgia, nicotine withdrawal, depression, chronic fatigue syndrome, hypothyroidism, or Rheumatoid Arthritis.

Some common symptoms associated with HPA dysfunction

Muscle Pain	Cold hands/legs	Dry skin
Headaches	Digestive problems	Dark circles under the eyes
Teeth grinding	Altered Appetite	

Another very important part of solving HPA dysfunction is understanding the part of the brain responsible for emotional firing: the limbic system. The limbic system is comprised of the amygdala, hippocampus, cingulate cortex, and hypothalamus.

Amygdala	Emotional memory like fear and anger
Hippocampus	Converting short-term memory into long-term memory

Cingulate Cortex	Memory, emotional processing, learning
Hypothalamus	Automatic regulator: blood pressure, hormones, temperature, metabolism, sexual arousal Links the mind-body connection[16]

Together some of the functions of the limbic system include sorting and filtering through sensory information and determining how we store, remember, and respond to it. This is the part of the brain that responds to threats in our environment. Normally it only fires when there is a real threat; however, in a dysfunctionally wired brain it may fire when it shouldn't. This has obvious deleterious cascading effects on the systems of our body. When the threat centers of the brain are activated, they send a stimulus to the hypothalamus to stimulate the adrenal glands to produce adrenaline. Every time you relive a bad memory this occurs and can become chronic. Personally, I was always in a state of thinking about my symptoms. The thought of whether my symptoms would flare up or cause discomfort or pain was always on my mind. This had me in a negative loop of firing stress signals.

The major pillars of stress effecting the HPA axis are gastrointestinal stress, circadian disruption, inflammatory signals, and perceived stress. I am going to spend the rest of the chapter talking about strategies for mitigating perceived stress.

If perceived stress has superiority over the HPA response then what influences perceived stress? There are different criteria that contribute to perceived stress including: the novelty of event, the unpredictability of an event, perceived threat to body or ego, a sense of loss of control, interpersonal relationships, public speaking, major road blocks of life goals, and violation of one's worldview. Are there ways to avoid making these stressors life-threatening hormonal events?

Dr. Bruce Lipton, a cell biologist who specialized in stem cell research for much of his career, expresses in his book, *Biology of Belief,* that it is the environment that causes disease and not our genetics. Throughout his experiments he discovered that when the nucleus of the cell was destroyed, the cell still continued to carry out metabolic processes for months with the one caveat of not being able to replicate. However, when you tamper with the cell membrane the cell dies immediately. The reason the cell does not die when the nucleus is destroyed is due to the receptors on the cell membrane that are given instructions via chemical messengers. These receptors are not limited to chemical messengers, but also react to light, sound, pressure, radio frequencies, and thousands of other environmental signals! This upgrades the cell membrane as the true "brain" of the cell, thereby downgrading the nucleus to being the cell gonads. This means if the cell membrane receptors are damaged by different stressors the cell is fighting an uphill battle even with proper nutrition. These findings suggest that genes do not control cell behavior, but rather are primarily crafted by the environment. This is tremendously empowering. Humans don't have that much bigger genomes than the most archaic bacteria on earth; however, our cell membranes have much greater surface area for hundreds of thousands of "switches" waiting to be activated/deactivated. Does this mean you can program your cells and yourself as an organism for health and prosperity? If you are feeding it the right signals, you bet!

Every immature cell in the human body has the same DNA. Signals from the environment determine how the cell will express itself and specialize. Epigenetics is the ability to turn genes off and on. Epigenetic expression can have up to 2,000+ protein variations for the same gene. Between 75–85 percent of genes can be manipulated by cell carrier pigeons, some in only a matter of seconds.[17] This means you can constantly level up to become the best version of yourself. It reminds me of Pokémon, except you can continue to evolve into better a version of you!

This brings me to the work of Dr. Joe Dispenza in *Breaking the Habit of Being You*. He talks about how our brains imprint memories of people, places, and things. Attached to each memory is an emotion. Every time you relive a memory associated with negative emotions, your body gets soaked in peptides and hormones associated with negative emotions turning on genes that prevent repair. When you have a thought or memory, electric and chemical signals are released in the brain. So quite literally your thoughts are matter. Over time, how you think becomes how you feel in a cycle. By the time you are 35, 95 percent of your thoughts are part of your unconscious wiring and only 5 percent are conscious. In order to override the program, you must spend time reprogramming yourself. This way your unconscious self produces appropriate thoughts for the production of beneficial chemicals to the body. We think between 60,000 to 70,000 thoughts a day, with over 90 percent of those thoughts being the same ones we had the day before.[18] Changing your thoughts is uncomfortable and expends energy. It is actually the biological, neurological, chemical, and even genetic death of your "old self." It only takes 3 weeks for neural connections to shrink, which is why you may commonly hear it takes 3 weeks to form a new habit.

> *"I'm never going to be healthy."*

> *"It's not fair that I have this disease."*

> *"Nobody cares."*

You can transform those thoughts into dirt roads, and turn:

> *"I am grateful for...."*

> *"I am so lucky for...."*

into frequently traveled highways in your brain.

A habit is a set of automatic, unconscious behaviors that you can teach your body to do. Repetition wires your body to do this. Changing to love, gratitude, and wholeness after decades of jealousy, frustration, and anger consuming your head is like trying to write with your less dominant hand; your body literally doesn't know how to do it.

If you continue to feed neurotransmitters to the neuronal cells of negative thought pathways over and over, it begins to expect and crave them. You literally become addicted to the thoughts that quench those receptors. No different than going into withdrawal from drug addiction. This may be why drama always finds one person and luck always finds another.

If you can stimulate digestive enzymes by thinking about food, or if you can get aroused by a simple daydream, then you can certainly turn on other gene expressions by thought alone. This means thinking positive, whether its real or not, can help facilitate healing instructions to cells. You cannot change the genetic expression until you change the signal to the cells.

When you're truly focused on an intention for some future outcome and you can make your inner thoughts more real than the outer environment during the process, the brain won't know the difference between the two. Then your body, as the unconscious mind, will begin to experience the new future event in the present moment. This will signal new genes in preparation for the newly imagined future event. Those same feelings of well-being influence you to make choices that bring you in that direction. These choices then become habits that create a cycle of thoughts and experiences that work for you.

You must constantly live in a future memory of yourself. A place where you have full health and you can feel the visceral excitement that goes along with having your health. These memories will bless yourself in neuropeptides and hormones that will stimulate repair genes to get you there! Studies tell us when you mentally rehearse a particular body part while elevating a positive emotion, you are activating the part of the brain that innervates that part of the body![19]

I applied the principals from Dr. Dispenza's work to myself, not only visualizing myself with full health every day during my meditation and reminding myself throughout the day, but I got granular with it. I pictured the ulcers in my intestines sealing up,

I pictured the hyperactive colon slowing down, my skin clearing, my joints bending like butter—and even giving lectures about my journey back to health. I would get up from the meditation in love with my body, health, and life, ready to conquer the day.

You, too, can devote 10 minutes a day to moving into an elevated state of joy, love, or gratitude. You can do it multiple times a day or for hours. The more the better!

When you feel safe and content, positive feelings cause a cascade that promotes more than 1,400 biochemical changes in the body for growth and repair. The chemical dump of well-being can last minutes.[20] The opposite is true when you are hurt, jealous, or angry. We are human and its ok to feel this way sometimes. In fact, psychological stress can also build resilience; however, we must be able to make sure these feelings are short-lived. If you let an event affect you for a few hours to a few days, the feeling turns into a mood. If you allow that event to affect you for weeks and months that mood turns into a temperament and if you allow it to change you for years it now becomes a personality trait. When you place your attention and awareness on your pain, it expands, because you experience more of it. Suffering from an autoimmune disease you have every reason to be mad, but what is extremely unreasonable is to allow it to make you mad because that contributes to the disease!

Researchers at Yale followed 660 people, aged 50 and older, for up to 23 years, discovering that those with a positive attitude about aging lived more than seven years longer than those who had a more negative outlook about growing older. Attitude had more of an influence on longevity than blood pressure, cholesterol levels, smoking, body weight, or level of exercise.[21]

To show the power of the mind-body connection further, 10 research subjects between the ages of 20 and 35 imagined flexing one of their biceps as hard as they could in 5 training sessions a week for 12 weeks. The researchers recorded the subjects' electrical brain activity and measured their muscle strength during the sessions, every other week. By the end of the study, the subjects had increased their biceps' strength by 13.5 percent, without ever touching a weight.[22]

Professional mindset coach Trevor Moawad shares that if someone says something out loud it is 10 times more powerful than if they think it. Negativity is a multiplier of 4–7 times that of positivity. So, if you say something out loud that is negative, it's a 40–70 times more likely that it will happen. If you can't think positive, at least think neutral.[23] You are not a professional athlete, but you are just as dedicated to your health as they are to the game and your mindset must reflect winning your health back. This illuminates the power of saying your daily affirmation, right after your eyes open to the world in the morning. "I, Colby Kash, am in robust health...."

I want to talk a little bit about what it means to meditate and what happens when you meditate. Most people are afraid to start because they don't know if they are "doing it right." The brain has different states of alertness that are defined by the frequency or wave that it fires electric signals. Your brain is in beta frequency when you are wired, active, alert, or anxious. Next comes the alpha brain wave whereby you are relaxed or analytical, but much of your focus is inward. The theta brain wave is a state of deep relaxation. Delta is the brain wave that you fall into during deep sleep and the state babies are in. Each of these brain waves exists within a range. So high beta is a lot different than low beta. In high beta, fight or flight, your programs are in control and you are more likely to say something you shouldn't have, or have a lapse in a bad habit you are trying to kick.

Human Brain Waves

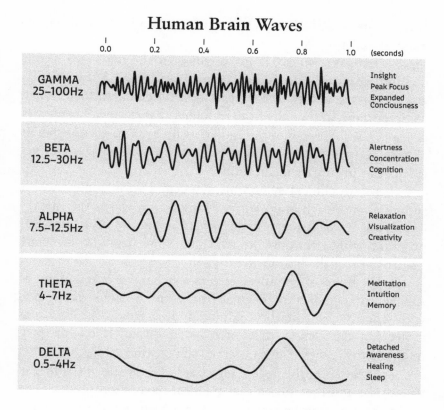

During a meditation, you put on headphones to hear soothing sounds or guidance that block the external world. You close your eyes to turn off more stimuli. Your brain can now calm down and lower into the alpha wave. While you are still aware of the outer world, the inner world becomes more real and attentive than the outer world. When your body falls asleep but your mind is awake, you have entered theta wave, a hypnotic state. Theta wave is the sweet spot for meditation. It is also possible to get into a fifth brain wave called gamma, which is the highest frequency. This deepest state of meditation is mixed with a profound surge of energy, increased perception of senses, and focus. Gamma waves are much more frequent among monks and experienced meditators. This state is also categorized by its ability to synchronize brain waves, so it's almost like all the brain regions are skipping rope at the same time.[24] There is still a lot more to be studied on this brain wave.

The mind is a "muscle." Just as you go to the gym to train your muscles, you meditate to gain control of the mind. Eventually, you obtain the ability to have calmness on demand, focus when it's important, and control the thoughts that deserve hospitality in your head. As the months and years fly by, you become better able to control the transition of brain waves, and you can get more done in shorter meditations.

There are clinical symptoms associated with dominance or suppression of each brain wave. Many turn towards the efficacy of EEG neurofeedback systems, which is the use of a computer program with electrodes attached to your head to stimulate homeostasis of the brain waves.

Just 8 hours of mindful meditation has been found to be sufficient to significantly change vital gene functions. Compared with controls, meditators exhibited a range of genetic and molecular differences that included reduced levels of pro-inflammatory genes. These observed changes in genetic expression are associated with faster physical recovery from stressful situations, and they prove that mindful meditation practice can lead to health improvement through epigenetic altercations of the genome.[25] In days, heart rate variability can change, followed by a modulation in the immune system. Although some benefits you may see right away, it takes years to become proficient.

The best time to do meditations are when you wake up and right before bed when you are closest to a state of theta wave dominance, but of course you will get benefits at any time of day. Personally, I enjoy Dr. Dispenza's guided meditations or Sam Harris's *Waking Up* app. I know it's not easy to think greater than you feel, but if you use your willpower tokens to change your habitual thoughts, once the exercise becomes a habit, you can use your new willpower tokens to form a new habit or stop a bad habit.

Meditation Sequence

Close your eyes and just focus on your breath; when your mind wanders to various problems, bring it back to focus on your breath.

I usually meditate 20 minutes in morning. I spend the first 10 minutes getting into a relaxed theta brain state and then the next 10 minutes plotting and creating my perfect life as though it exists in the now. The more I do this, the more I strengthen the neurocircuits in my brain, while breaking the ones that I don't want in my future.

The mindset is not to pray for something, but to get up from the meditation with your prayers already answered.

Throughout the rest of the day, when that negative predicted negative thought comes to you, simply become aware of it and remember what you practiced in the meditation.

One added bonus occurs if you hum during the meditation. Humming increases nitric oxide up to 15 times in the nasal passages, which can effectively open the airways.[26]

In *Wired for Healing,* Annie Hopper describes 12 steps she used to heal her dysfunctional limbic system that was contributing to her chemical and environmental sensitivities that forced her to become homeless. Her approach includes principles from both Dr. Dispeza and Dr. Lipton and adds an algorithmic flow to follow.

The steps are:

- Develop awareness of dysfunction in the limbic system: physical, psychological, emotional, or behavioral patterns;

- Recognize and diagnose these symptoms as limbic system dysfunction;

- Interrupt the patterns associated with limbic dysfunction;

- Decrease fear association to stimuli;

- Reattribute symptoms to over-activated threat mechanism;

- Choose a new strategy for responding to stimuli;

- Cultivate a positive emotional state to diminish stress response;

- Cultivate a positive psychological state to restrain thought patterns associated with catastrophic thinking;

- Incrementally train yourself to strengthen new brain pathways and desensitize triggers;

- Change habits associated with extreme harm-avoidance behaviors;

- Recognize improvements and celebrate them;

- Repeat the new strategy daily for a minimum of an hour for 6 months.[27]

Another unique conundrum of modern humanity is loneliness. For most of human history, we lived-in close-knit tribes, and in more modern times families lived in tight social multigenerational households, which was very common up to 50 years ago. In the industrialized world this has declined due to schooling and job opportunities. The safety net of the multigenerational household provided social support in times of stress, a sort of mental floss against depression and anxiety. Just like a muscle, relationships atrophy if you don't nurture them. It is incumbent upon you to make the effort to stay in touch.

An 80-year longitudinal study from Harvard found that the happiest people later in life had one thing in common: they nurtured and preserved lifelong relationships with friends and family. Those strong relationships protect people from life's deteriorations by delaying mental and physical decline and are better predictors of long and happy lives than social class, IQ, or even genes.[28] Lonely and non-lonely people show different gene expression in 209 genes, many which play roles in inflammatory immune responses.[29] It is very easy while you are suffering from the pains or embarrassments of autoimmunity to retreat away from others. However, you need the social support more than ever and you must make time for social interactions like you would for the gym or meditation. I understand that many individuals who are isolated are not always so by choice. Proactive measures must be taken to join clubs or classes, to volunteer, using meet up apps/websites, and various other activities.

Oxytocin is regarded as the love hormone and gets released when you bond with friends and family, hug someone, practice gratitude, or in very high amounts when a mother births her child. The intestines and immune system organs have oxytocin receptors. When the oxytocin binds to white blood cells it turns off the production of inflammatory signals.[30] This hormone has been linked to modulating the immune system and down regulates the HPA axis.[31]

Those who volunteer have lower rates of depression, and this is especially true in people who are 65 and older. One to two hours a week of volunteering is the amount that's been shown to be required for significant health benefits.[32] Volunteering is a fantastic option because it not only increases social support but provides a sense of purpose, which is also very important to health and well-being. Interestingly, studies have found interpersonal stressors such as social humiliation and damaged reputation are amongst the strongest predictors of emotional distress, systemic inflammation, poor health, and survival.[33, 34] This illuminates the importance of surrounding yourself with the right team and eliminating the toxic people in your life. Another effective strategy is getting an emotional support animal.

People who hold more spiritual or religious beliefs have significantly better mental health and adapt more quickly to health problems than those who are less spiritual. Perhaps, this is because of the community that surrounds them. Spiritual belief has a positive influence on the immune and endocrine systems. Having a strong faith can re-establish a sense of belonging and provides a sense of purpose, hope, and meaning in life despite negative experiences. In fact, those believing in something greater than themselves have lower infection rates and fewer stress hormones, as well as higher functioning white blood cells than non-spiritual patients.[35] My goal here is not to promote any particular type of religion, faith, or spiritual practice, but I think the overarching idea here is that having a broader perspective that expands beyond yourself is an important aspect of mental health.

Miscellaneous Tips

I don't think the healing phase is the time to conquer your fear of heights or public speaking. You do not need the extra stressor in your life. By all means once you get your autoimmune disease under control you can and should conquer these fears.

Although caffeine has some health benefits, and 1–2 cups of coffee are fine if tolerated, having too many cups a day produces stress hormones and will add to the stress load you are trying to minimize.

You only want beneficial chemical messengers bathing your cells. This may mean cleansing yourself of brain junk food like the news, scary movies and shows. Silence the posts and stories of certain people on social media. This may be tough at first while you break your addiction to those chemicals. Switch to funny upbeat and inspirational entertainment.

Take relaxing movement meditation breaks—like Qigong or Tai chi—throughout the day to regain your composure and take control of your thoughts.

Taking control of the mind is a major pillar to reversing your autoimmune disease and increasing quality of life. Dysfunctional hormonal patterns must be addressed and treated. The strategies discussed in the chapter should be gradually applied into your daily routine and tailored to what works best for you.

NOTES

1   McCorry, L. K. (2007, Aug. 15). *Physiology of the autonomic nervous system*. American journal of pharmaceutical education. Retrieved from https://www.ncbi.nlm.nih.gov/pmc/articles/PMC1959222.

2   Tsigos, C. (2020, Oct. 17). *Stress: Endocrine physiology and pathophysiology*. Endotext [Internet]. Retrieved from https://www.ncbi.nlm.nih.gov/books/NBK278995.

3   *An overview of the hypothalamus*. EndocrineWeb. Retrieved from https://www.endocrineweb.com/endocrinology/overview-hypothalamus.

4   *An overview of the pituitary gland*. EndocrineWeb. (n.d.). Retrieved from https://www.endocrineweb.com/endocrinology/overview-pituitary-gland.

5   *The sympathoadrenal system | SpringerLink*. Retrieved from https://link.springer.com/chapter/10.1007/978-1-4684-2502-4_10.

6   *Hypocortisolism: An evidence-based review - a4m.com*. (n.d.). Retrieved from https://www.a4m.com/assets/pdf/IntResources1IMCJ_10_4_p26-33_Hypocortisolism_3.pdf.

7   Slominski, A., Zbytek, B., Zmijewski, M., Slominski, R. M., Kauser, S., Wortsman, J., & Tobin, D. J. (2006, September 1). *Corticotropin releasing hormone and the skin*. Frontiers in bioscience : a journal and virtual library. Retrieved from https://www.ncbi.nlm.nih.gov/pmc/articles/PMC1847336.

8   *The ratio of DHEA or DHEA-S to cortisol - tahoma clinic*. (n.d.). Retrieved from https://tahomaclinic.com/Research/HandbookPDFs/DHEA-Cortisol-Ratio.pdf.

9   Rendina, D. N.; Ryff, C. D.; Coe, C. L. (2017, June 1). *Precipitous dehydroepiandrosterone declines reflect decreased physical vitality and function*. The journals of gerontology. Series A, Biological sciences and medical sciences. Retrieved from https://www.ncbi.nlm.nih.gov/pmc/articles/PMC6074872.

10 Roy, S.; Khanna, S.; Yeh, P. E.; Rink, C.; Malarkey, W. B.; Kiecolt-Glaser, J.; Laskowski, B.; Glaser, R.; Sen, C. K. (n.d.). *Wound site neutrophil transcriptome in response to psychological stress in young men*. Gene expression. Retrieved from https://pubmed.ncbi.nlm.nih.gov/16358416.

11 *DHEA modulates immune function: A review of evidence . . .* (n.d.). Retrieved from https://www.researchgate.net/publication/323671578_DHEA_Modulates_Immune_Function_A_Review_of_Evidence.

12 Cohen, S.; Janicki-Deverts, D.; Doyle, W. J.; Miller, G. E.; Frank, E.; Rabin, B. S.; Turner, R. B. (2012, April 17). *Chronic stress, glucocorticoid receptor resistance, inflammation, and disease risk*. Proceedings of the National Academy of Sciences of the United States of America. Retrieved from https://www.ncbi.nlm.nih.gov/pmc/articles/PMC3341031.

13   Chetty, S.; Friedman, A. R.; Taravosh-Lahn, K.; Kirby, E. D.; Mirescu, C.;
     Guo, F.; Krupik, D.; Nicholas, A.; Geraghty, A.; Krishnamurthy, A.; Tsai,
     M. K.; Covarrubias, D.; Wong, A.; Francis, D.; Sapolsky, R. M.; Palmer,
     T. D.; Pleasure, D.; Kaufer, D. (n.d.). *Stress and glucocorticoids promote
     oligodendrogenesis in the adult hippocampus.* Molecular psychiatry.
     Retrieved from https://pubmed.ncbi.nlm.nih.gov/24514565.

14   Silverman, M. N. and Sternberg, E. M. (2012, July). *Glucocorticoid
     regulation of inflammation and its functional correlates: From HPA axis
     to glucocorticoid receptor dysfunction.* Annals of the New York Academy
     of Sciences. Retrieved from https://www.ncbi.nlm.nih.gov/pmc/articles/
     PMC3572859.

15   Broersen, L. H. A.; Pereira, A. M.; Jørgensen, J. O. L.; Dekkers, O. M.
     (2015, June 1). *Adrenal insufficiency in corticosteroids use: Systematic
     review and meta-analysis.* OUP Academic. Retrieved from https://academic.
     oup.com/jcem/article/100/6/2171/2829580.

16   Rajmohan, V. and Mohandas, E. (2007, April). *The limbic system.* Indian
     journal of psychiatry. Retrieved from https://www.ncbi.nlm.nih.gov/pmc/
     articles/PMC2917081.

17   Lipton, B. H. (2003). *The Biology of Belief.* Spirit 2000, Inc.

     Dispenza, J. and Amen, D. G. (2015). *Breaking the habit of being yourself:
     How to lose your mind and create a new one.* Hay House.

18   Dispenza, J. and Amen, D. G. (2015). *Breaking the habit of being yourself:
     How to lose your mind and create a new one.* Hay House.

19   E;, E. H. H. G. S. N. (n.d.). *Imagery of voluntary movement of fingers,
     toes, and tongue activates corresponding body-part-specific motor
     representations.* Journal of neurophysiology. Retrieved from https://
     pubmed.ncbi.nlm.nih.gov/14615433.

20   Dispenza, J. and Amen, D. G. (2015). *Breaking the habit of being yourself:*
     ...

21   SV;, L. B. R. S. M. D. K. S. R. K. (n.d.). *Longevity increased by positive
     self-perceptions of aging.* Journal of personality and social psychology.
     Retrieved from https://pubmed.ncbi.nlm.nih.gov/12150226.

22   Cohen, P. "Mental Gymnastics Increase Bicep Strength." *New Scientist,*
     vol. 172, no. 2318: p. 17 (2001). http://www.newscientist.com/article
     /dn1591-mental-gymnastics-increase-bicep-strength.html#.Ui03PLzk_V

23   YouTube. (2020, March 3). *Mindset expert shows you how to control your
     negative thoughts | trevor moawad on impact theory.* YouTube. Retrieved
     from   https://www.youtube.com/watch?v=5lCeWtXPKko&feature=emb_
     title.

24   *Gamma wave.* Gamma Wave—an overview | ScienceDirect Topics.
     (n.d.). Retrieved from https://www.sciencedirect.com/topics/neuroscience/
     gamma-wave.

25   Kaliman, P.; Alvarez-López, M. J.; Cosín-Tomás, M.; Rosenkranz, M.
     A.; Lutz, A.; Davidson, R. J. (2014, Feb.). *Rapid changes in histone
     deacetylases and inflammatory gene expression in expert meditators.*

Psychoneuroendocrinology. Retrieved from https://www.ncbi.nlm.nih.gov/pmc/articles/PMC4039194.

26 GA;, E. (n.d.). *Strong humming for one hour daily to terminate chronic rhinosinusitis in four days: A case report and hypothesis for action by stimulation of endogenous nasal nitric oxide production.* Medical hypotheses. Retrieved from https://pubmed.ncbi.nlm.nih.gov/16406689.

27 Hopper, A. (2014). *Wired for healing: Remapping the brain to recover from chronic amysteriousous illnesses.* The Dynamic Neural Retraining System.

28 Mineo, L. (2018, Nov.). *Over nearly 80 years, Harvard study has been showing how to live a healthy and happy life.* Harvard Gazette. Retrieved from https://news.harvard.edu/gazette/story/2017/04/over-nearly-80-years -harvard-study-has-been-showing-how-to-live-a-healthy-and-happy-life.

29 Cole, S. W. (2009, June 1). *Social Regulation of human gene expression.* Current directions in psychological science. Retrieved from https://www.ncbi.nlm.nih.gov/pmc/articles/PMC3020789.

30 Szeto, A.; Nation, D. A.; Mendez, A. J.; Dominguez-Bendala, J.; Brooks, L. G.; Schneiderman, N.; McCabe, P. M. (n.d.). *Oxytocin attenuates NADPH-dependent superoxide activity and IL-6 secretion in macrophages and vascular cells.* American journal of physiology. Endocrinology and metabolism. Retrieved from https://pubmed.ncbi.nlm.nih.gov/18940936.

31 Clodi, M.; Vila, G.; Geyeregger, R.; Riedl, M.; Stulnig, T. M.; Struck, J.; Luger, T. A.; Luger, A. (n.d.). *Oxytocin alleviates the neuroendocrine and cytokine response to bacterial endotoxin in Healthy Men.* American journal of physiology. Endocrinology and metabolism. from https://pubmed.ncbi.nlm.nih.gov/18593851.

32 The Journals of Gerontology. (2018, March). *Does Becoming A Volunteer Attenuate Loneliness Among Recently Widowed Older Adults?* Oxford Academic. Retrieved from https://academic.oup.com/psychsocgerontology/article/73/3/501/3938841?login=true.

33 Seeman, M.; Stein Merkin, S.; Karlamangla, A.; Koretz, B.; Seeman, T. (2014, Oct.). *Social status and biological dysregulation: The "status syndrome" and Allostatic Load.* Social science & medicine (1982). Retrieved from https://www.ncbi.nlm.nih.gov/pmc/articles/PMC4167677.

34 Epel, E. S.; Crosswell, A. D.; Mayer, S. E.; Prather, A. A.; Slavich, G. M.; Puterman, E.; Mendes, W. B. (2018, April). *More than a feeling: A unified view of stress measurement for population science.* Frontiers in neuroendocrinology. Retrieved from https://www.ncbi.nlm.nih.gov/pmc/articles/PMC6345505.

35 Koenig, H. G. (2012, Dec. 16). *Religion, spirituality, and Health: The Research and Clinical Implications.* ISRN psychiatry. Retrieved from https://www.ncbi.nlm.nih.gov/pmc/articles/PMC3671693.

CHAPTER 6

Sleep

SUDDENLY, MY EYES AWOKE, but my body did not follow. As I lay motionless, it occurred to me that my body was paralyzed, and a warm coat of anxiety rushed through me. After about 30 seconds my body was freed. This was my first experience with sleep paralysis and was well-deserved. I had been studying abroad in beautiful, medieval Florence, Italy. I had not taken a single night off from living young, wild, and free, followed by early morning ringtones of *Love Generations* from my alarm clock, alerting me that it was time to get up for class. Sleep paralysis is a trippy neurologic experience when you transiently cannot move your limbs, cannot speak, and for some people, cannot open up their eyes.[1] And it is certainly a sign you are not giving your body and brain the proper recovery needed.

I had hacked into the wonders of sleep deprivation a few other times in my life, once while pledging a fraternity when we were forced to stay awake for 48 hours while being ordered to sort candy sprinkles, wrestle on concrete, and listen to the same song on repeat for hours. I remember hallucinating and being unaware of my whereabouts. I knew where I was, but I didn't know where I was was. Another experience I had was when I participated in a dance marathon and we "danced" for 26.2 hours to raise money for the Children's Miracle Network. Boy, the body felt that for a few days.

Aside from these extreme examples, I always made it a priority to get 8 hours of sleep a night. I now know that even frequent small amounts of sleep deprivation each night put a strain on your stress bank. This chapter explores the consequences of inefficient sleep on the immune system, and how we can optimize sleep.

Between 50–70 million Americans suffer from chronic long-term sleep disorders, which are associated with major depression, anxiety, suicidal behavior, and autoimmune disease.[2] This is largely because when we sleep, our brains get much needed rest and rejuvenation. As the Greek poet Archilochus of Paros (ca. 680–640 BC) wrote, "recognize which rhythms govern man." Over 2,500 years later, we now know that biological rhythms govern immense aspects of human behavior, physiology, metabolism, disease symptoms, and response to treatment in a cycle called circadian rhythm.[3]

The circadian rhythm is a natural internal clock that regulates the sleep-wake cycle that repeats approximately every 24 hours. It responds to light, temperature, food availability, and it might have a seasonal component as well. Homeostasis is maintained in the body through a large number of bidirectional interactions among physiological systems. The circadian and immune systems play leading roles in this dynamic behavior, and their effective regulation is of utmost importance. Experimental evidence shows that chronically stressful conditions often disturb the rhythmic orchestration of the body, resulting in the blunting of critical endocrine signals. The circadian rhythm controls hundreds of synchronized systems in the body, including body temperature, metabolic rate, grip strength, and your mental state.

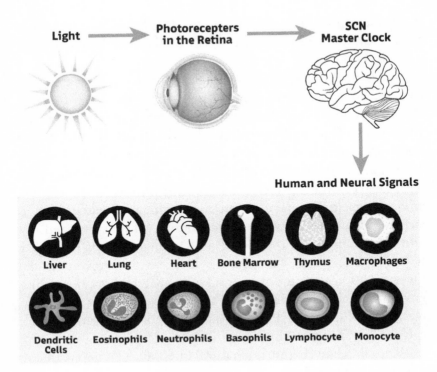

Light stimulates specialized cells in the eyes that transmit the signal to command central, the hypothalamus. The hypothalamus, the body's grandfather clock, is responsible for synchronizing the many simultaneous systematic rhythms of the human body. Tens of thousands of nerve cells emanate from the hypothalamus to relay the signal to the body's moving parts.

As explained in Chapter 5, the hypothalamus is the major control tower of all hormone production in the body and the governor of the stress response. The part of the hypothalamus that's responsible for the body's circadian rhythm is called the superchiasmatic nucleus, or SCN. This puts the SCN in control of many genes, including immune function and pain sensitivity. The SCN is fully formed by the time we are 3–4 years old, thereby beginning to obey the circadian rhythm as we move from polyphasic naps to biphasic or monophasic sleep cycles.

The SCN is stimulated by light exposure and the Earth's 24-hour light-dark cycle. This means that artificial light, especially blue light, stimulates the SCN at night, thereby promoting cortisol release and causing an inhibition of melatonin as the two hormones work contrary to each other. Melatonin is the hormone that sets the stage for sleep. While the right amount of blue light during the day, especially in the morning, is beneficial, when the sun goes down, blue light becomes a toxic stressor and bounces the body out of homeostasis. Once again, cortisol is not secreted in a uniform amount throughout the day, but rather in a diurnal fashion, so the highest levels of cortisol would be produced around 8:00 a.m., after which there is a gradual decline throughout the day until between midnight and 4:00 a.m. Then it rises again quickly, resulting in peak output just as we are waking up. This explains why telling your body it is daytime at nighttime is a major disrupter to the HPA axis.

Circadian discombobulation leads to dysregulation of immune responses and inflammation, which can further disrupt circadian rhythms. There is considerable bidirectional interaction between sleep and the immune system. The immune system cells peak during certain times and dip during others. A reduction in sleep below 5 hours per night correlates with an increased risk of common cold, pneumonia, and altered allergic reactions.[4, 5] One theory even suggests that our immune system has evolved to deal with different pathogens at their most likely times of infection, thereby causing a cycle of our white blood cell numbers. The circadian secretion of melatonin also plays a role in regulating the expression of immune-mediating cytokines. Melatonin is released from the pineal gland in the brain and has a strong immunomodulatory impact and the ability to decrease TNF.[6] In cases where the pineal gland has to be removed, immune complications—consisting of sophisticated feedback loops that function in immune synchrony—will follow.

Sleep is necessary to make your gut happy. When you do not get enough sleep, the body's stress-related, fight-or-flight nervous system revs up, triggering an excess of circulating cortisol that cultivates "bad bacteria." As a result, insufficient sleep will prevent the meaningful absorption of all food nutrients and can lead to gastrointestinal problems. Lack of sleep allows the toxins from intestinal bacteria such as lipopolysaccharides to cross the gut barrier, which increases cytokines and TNF systematically.[7] Cytokines in the gut cascade to the brain; brain inflammation is going to fragment sleep. This becomes a vicious cycle of lack of sleep increasing cytokines, and cytokines causing lack of sleep. Specifically, when studied in autoimmune disease, chronic lack of adequate sleep accelerates the onset of Lupus.[8] How can you possibly recover from a complex autoimmune in such an immune frenzy?

One study found that sleep deprivation led to an invasion of pathogenic bacteria into normally sterile body tissues. In fact, the evidence reveals that the cause of death in those with chronic sleep deprivation is bacteria translocation in the gut.[9] In other words, the inability to fend off innocuous communal infections on the skin and in the gut kills you! A single night of 4 hours of sleep swept away 70 percent of the natural killer cells that circulate in the immune system, when compared to a full eight-hour night of sleep. That is a dramatic state of immune deficiency that can happen after a single bad night of sleep. Consistently sleeping less than 6 or 7 hours a night chronically obliterates the immune system. Two-thirds of adults in Western industrialized societies do not get the recommended 8 hours of sleep every night. After 10 days of just 7 hours of sleep a night, the brain is as dysfunctional as it would be after going without sleep for 24 hours. Even three full nights of recovery sleep are insufficient to restore performance back to normal levels after a week of poor sleep patterns.

The circadian cycle is meant to be obeyed at the same time every day. Even if you go to bed 2 hours later on the weekend or on any particular night, you are going to miss out on most of the deep sleep that the body experiences during the beginning of the sleep cycle. And deep sleep is when you get a huge boost in growth hormone release, which is responsible for rebuilding your gut and joint linings. Brain scans of individuals who are sleep-deprived have higher reactivity in the fear centers of the brain when viewing the same images as the control group. Without sleep, our brain reverts to a primitive pattern of uncontrolled reactivity. This explains the cranky phenomenon. The less sleep, the less willpower you will have to make the strong food choices, the strong habitual changes you will need to make on your journey back to health. Now let's say you are good about going to bed the same time every night, but you only allow for 6 hours of sleep. Waking up just 2 hours early can cause you to miss a significant amount of REM (rapid eye movement) sleep. This stage of sleep is when you experience dreaming. REM sleep converts memories with emotions attached to it, into long-term storage.

After one week of reduced sleep in mice, the activities of 711 genes were distorted, relative to their normal sleep schedule. The genes that were turned on included those linked to chronic inflammation, cellular stress, various factors that cause cardiovascular disease, and the genes that help maintain stable metabolism and optimal immune responses were downregulated.[10] Neglecting sleep effectively genetically engineers your body into poor health.

Maybe you make ample time for sleep and put it high on your priority list, but you just can't fall asleep. The two most common triggers of chronic insomnia are psychological worries and anxiety. In this fast-paced, information-overloaded modern world, one of the few times that we stop our persistent informational consumption and inwardly reflect is when our heads hit the pillow. There is no worse time to consciously do this. (Ways to mitigate psychological stress were addressed in Chapter 5.)

If we are expected to give up 25–30 years of our lives for sleeping, it had better pay its dividends. You bet it does! It's not just time in bed that counts, but sleep latency, amount of deep sleep, and REM sleep. Quality sleep allows you to become the best version of yourself in mood, performance, or health. Knowing this, you should make it an uncompromising mission to become an expert on sleep. The sleep strategies that are shared later in the chapter have the most profound effects when used in parallel.

Is it worth breaking bedtime to watch another episode of that show? To stay up late texting? To be at the club till 4:00 a.m.? The answers to those questions during the healing phase are a resounding NO. These are the sacrifices you must make to heal. Love yourself enough to make the sacrifices. Then, as you begin to feel better, you can "reintroduce" late nights for special events where you stay up for social gatherings and so forth.

Shift Work

The unnatural work shifts in a 24/7 work week were popularized in the late 1800s with the invention of artificial light, which progressed to TVs and, in more recent decades, the advent of cellphones, computers, and other devices. Nurses, doctors, EMTs, computer operators, many within the air travel profession, and protective services personnel, all sacrifice their natural biological systems. About 3 percent of the workforce in industrialized nations take on the graveyard shift.[11] I feel very blessed that there are so many members of society willing to make this sacrifice. However, the chronic disruption of the body's physiology leads to some unfortunate side effects, as their day begins when the body prepares to relax the systems by decreasing core body temperature, alertness, and performance. It is commonly reported that night-shift workers endure shortened daytime sleep and are increasingly sleepy during awake hours.

Those who are on a consistent night shift every day may be able to adapt somewhat, but an alternating shift is just a complete disaster for the HPA axis. Studies show that the most taxing shift work is where workers work the night shift twice a week and then a day shift 2–3 days a week. This allows for no sort of adaptation.[12] Perhaps some policy change would allow for the health protection of police officers and emergency medical services to move to more consistent shifts.

Shift work is significantly correlated with increased rates of Autoimmune Thyroid disease[13] and Rheumatoid Arthritis.[14] The Rheumatoid Arthritis inflammatory markers were the worst with alternating day/night shifts. Diseases such as obesity, diabetes, viral infections, gastrointestinal issues, and cardiovascular disease are more common among shift workers.[15] As a result, there may be a relationship between circadian rhythmicity and disease development. When was the last time you got a prescription to simply "sleep" from your doctor?

Jet Lag

Jet lag is yet another modern phenomenon that alters the natural circadian clock. It generally takes one day per hour of time change for adaptation to the time zone. For frequent business travelers this can keep your body in an endocrine guessing game. On top of the time zone, if you're taking a red-eye flight, you are getting poor sleep while getting bombarded by radiation—all of which adds up to a triple whammy.

Scientists have studied airplane cabin crews who frequently fly on long-haul routes and have little chance to recover. Two alarming results have emerged. First, parts of their brains, specifically those related to learning and memory, had physically shrunk. This suggests the destruction of brain cells. Second, their short-term memory was significantly impaired. They were considerably more forgetful than individuals of similar age and background who did not frequently travel through time zones. Other studies of pilots, cabin crew members, and shift workers have reported additionally disquieting consequences, including far higher rates of cancer and Type 2 Diabetes than among the general population.[16]

Another factor in frequent travel is not sleeping at home. When you're traveling, your bedtime routine is going to be disrupted and you won't be as comfortable. Reports suggest that humans have a mild version of unihemispheric sleep, similar to the way dolphins or birds sleep with one hemisphere of the brain at a time. When a person is brought into a sleep laboratory or taken to a hotel, one half of the brain sleeps a little more lightly than the other, almost as if standing guard for protection. The more nights an individual sleeps in the new location, the more similar the sleep is in each half of the brain. It is the reason why so many of us sleep poorly when we're "on the road."[17]

For those who try and make up for their sleep deficit on the weekend, they are simply flirting with rest and recovery. After three nights of ample sleep, performance still does not return to baseline.[18] The brain is unable to bounce back like we wish it would. This is referred to as social jet lag, as you start Monday with your circadian rhythm pushed several hours later.

Similar to shift work, jet lag pays such a taxing effect on the body's natural circadian system that it may give you second thoughts about your career if you are suffering from autoimmunity. I understand this is not an easy decision, but I run on the premise that your health and the ability to thrive and reach your full potential are of utmost importance. During the healing phase, consider it. Before having that conversation, there are also "hacks" available to mitigate the effects.

How to mitigate the effects of jet lag

- Try and get a lot of bright light around the time you are setting the body to wake up. There is device called a re-timer, which actually are glasses that feature a wavelength of light emanating from underneath, thus simulating daylight. Using this when you wake will simulate daytime. Humans have photoreceptors in our ears, so another device that acts to simulate daytime is called the "human charger," and it shines blue light into your ears. You can wear it like headphones.

- Cold exposure such as a cold shower shortly after rising can shift your circadian earlier.

- Exercising shortly after rising can shift your circadian earlier.

- Do not eat for several hours before bed.

- Towards the end of your shift, you can wear blue-blocking glasses and use blue light filters on computers/phones to prevent the melatonin inhibition from blue/bright lights.

Sleep Hacks

The hours leading to bed have a significant effect on sleep, as neurotransmitters and hormones start to change concentration. Our ancestors would have not struggled with this natural process; however, in 21st-century Western society we have the blessing and curse of artificial light. As we learned earlier in the chapter, artificial blue lights inhibit our bodies' melatonin production. Blue light-blocking glasses can filter the harmful wavelength waging war on your sleep. The slightest amount of light, just 8 lux, has been shown to inhibit the release of melatonin production by 50 percent. Bedside lamps can be from 20–80 lux and a lit room can be 200 lux, which is only 1–2 percent of daylight.[19] Reading from an iPad before bed, even when it's turned to night mode, significantly decreases melatonin production. This has a cascading effect of less deep sleep, REM sleep, and an increase in daytime sleepiness.[20]

Sleep Hygiene Strategies

- Swap bright white light bulbs to bulbs that do not have the blue wavelength of light. I personally like red lights. Another tip is not to have beaming overhead lights that simulate daylight, but rather lower lights to simulate a red hue as if from a campfire.

- The most important strategy is keeping a strict bedtime. Go to bed and wake up at the same time each day. As creatures of habit, people have a hard time adjusting to changes in sleep patterns. This will prevent social jet lag.

- The bedroom should be completely blacked out. Blackout shades should be used, and light from any devices should be turned off. Also, you can use eye shades, which are great while traveling.

- Electric stimulation can help stimulate sleep. There is a current referred to as microcurrent, which runs at the same physiologic frequency as your cells so you don't generally feel it when it's placed on skin. When that current is run intracranially via ear clips, it stimulates the pineal gland to produce serotonin. Serotonin is a deficient neurotransmitter in those with insomnia. Serotonin is a precursor to the production of melatonin. At the same time, it inhibits acetylcholine, a neurotransmitter responsible for alertness and wakefulness. When microcurrent is used in this fashion, it is referred to as alpha stimulation. This is an FDA-cleared treatment for insomnia, anxiety, and depression. The treatment lasts 20–60 minutes. Just throw those bad boys on while reading and winding down before bed. Over time, you can decrease the frequency of treatment. There are no serious side effects aside from potential light-headedness or tingles. Specific research in Fibromyalgia patients saw a significant decrease in sleep disturbance.[21]

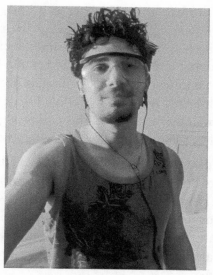

Here is a picture of me before bed, with my blue light blockers, red light bulb, and alpha stimulation.

- Keep a worry journal where you can list any concerns or responsibilities that are on your mind.

- Gravity blanket: Weighted blankets weigh between 5–30 pounds. The weighted pressure mimics hands-on pressure, thereby relaxing the nervous system. Studies have shown that gravity blankets reduce the time it took to fall asleep and the number of times sleep was disrupted during the night in those with anxiety.[22]

- To match the natural simulation of sunrise and sunset, your body's temperature drops in the evening, which helps initiate melatonin production. The external signals for melatonin production are not just light but also temperature. The human body actively participates in the lowering of its temperature. In order to shed heat, the body brings blood to the skin surface area, mostly in the hands, feet, and head where there is a tremendous amount of vascular surface area. They act as a body ventilation system. Lowering the thermostat in the room was a significant way my deep sleep times increased. The ideal sleeping temperature is between 60–67°F. There are some unique cooling technologies out there. One is the Chilipad, which flows cooled water through a mat from underneath you. This can be a great way to personalize temperature if you sleep with a partner.

- Do not exercise 2 hours before your bedtime. It can raise core body temperature too high, which will turn on the sympathetic nervous system. Even playing ping-pong too close to bedtime will drive up your heart rate and will keep you lying awake longer. Participate in relaxing activities.

- Don't take naps later in the afternoon. Naps can help make up for lost sleep, but late afternoon naps can make it harder to fall asleep at night. You should ideally take your nap when you are the least alert, which is typically 7–8 hours after you wake.

- Leave your cell phone on other side of room.

- Don't lie in bed awake. If you find yourself still awake after staying in bed for more than 20 minutes, or if you are starting to feel anxious or worried, get up and do a relaxing activity until you feel sleepy. The anxiety of not being able to sleep can make it harder to fall asleep.

- Invest in comfortable pillow/mattress.

- Orgasming with a partner is associated with better sleep outcomes. Masturbation is also correlated to better sleep outcomes but not as strongly. This is likely explained by the release of oxytocin, the love hormone, which has been shown to promote sleep.[23]

- Noise canceler: I use a few different tools to block out noise, depending on where I am sleeping. These include the sonic sleep app, a white noise machine, or a head band with flat earphones from sleepphones.com.

Quantification Devices

The importance of sleep should be an extraordinarily high priority for you and should be tracked no differently than blood pressure or cholesterol. There are various wearable devices that track many markers of sleep, including the different sleep stages (NREM, REM), how long it takes to fall asleep, how many times you moved in the night, and how sleep-efficient you were. This is a great tool to learn how adding and taking away various external stimuli affects your sleep.

I learned a lot of information about my sleep by wearing a sleep-tracking device. One thing that really shocked me was that having even one glass of wine close to bedtime decreased deep sleep by 75 percent. However, having a drink earlier in the evening did not have much of an effect on deep sleep. When you drink, many people knock out very easily; however, this is not restorative deep sleep, and you will wake up groggy. Alcohol is a strong inhibitor of the quality sleep you need. Furthermore, it bombards the GABA receptors, causing an overstimulation effect that wears off, causing you to wake up in the middle of the night, and makes it hard to fall back asleep.

Food, Drinks, and
Supplements Related to Sleep

A neurotransmitter called adenosine builds up in your brain throughout the day. It is responsible for the "sleep pressure," making it hard to keep your eyes open. The longer you are awake, the more adenosine will accumulate. Eventually, adenosine concentrations peak, and an irresistible urge to snooze takes over. Caffeine binds to the same receptors as adenosine in the brain. It effectively blocks them from adenosine, diminishing the sleep pressure. Caffeine has a half-life of 5–7 hours. This means if you have a cup of coffee at 5:00 p.m., by 12:00 a.m. you may still have 50 percent of the caffeine in your system. This is clearly going to have deleterious effects on your sleep. It is also worth noting that decaffeinated coffee can have 15–30 percent of the caffeine in a normal cup of coffee. There is some variability in how fast individuals break down caffeine; some are fast oxidizers while others like myself are slow oxidizers and caffeine will linger much longer.[24, 25]

Melatonin doesn't regulate sleep alone. It sends messages to other parts of the body in preparation for sleep, including the pancreas, where it binds to receptors and signals the temporary suppression of insulin production. This wasn't a problem in our pre-industrial past, but in today's environment of 24-hour food availability, it can have far-reaching effects on health. Increased levels of insulin can inhibit melatonin production.[26] You should avoid consumption of food 3–4 hours before bedtime.

Drinking too many fluids at night can cause frequent awakenings to urinate.

Sleep supplements that have been shown to increase sleep latency and deep sleep include

Magnesium Glycinate	L-theanine
Zinc	CBD

In today's world we must use technology to our advantage to reinstate quality sleep in order to heal our bodies. This includes engineering a sleep environment with the right amount of light, temperature, and comfort. When these signals fall into place so will our immune system, circadian rhythm, and the homeostatic nature our bodies are meant to be in.

NOTES

1   G. Browne Goode, M. (1962, March 1). *Sleep paralysis.* Archives of Neurology. Retrieved from https://jamanetwork.com/journals/jamaneurology/article-abstract/563685.

2   Colten, H. R. (1970, Jan. 1). *Extent and health consequences of chronic sleep loss and sleep disorders.* Sleep Disorders and Sleep Deprivation: An Unmet Public Health Problem. Retrieved from https://www.ncbi.nlm.nih.gov/books/NBK19961.

3   Comas, M.; Gordon, C. J.; Oliver, B. G.; Stow, N. W.; King, G.; Sharma, P.; Ammit, A. J.; Grunstein, R. R.; Phillips, C. L. (2017, Sept. 25). *A circadian based inflammatory response – implications for respiratory disease and treatment.* Sleep Science and Practice. Retrieved from https://link.springer.com/article/10.1186/s41606-017-0019-2.

4   Christ, P.; Sowa, A. S.; Froy, O.; Lorentz, A. (2018, July 6). *The circadian clock drives mast cell functions in allergic reactions.* Frontiers in immunology. Retrieved from https://www.ncbi.nlm.nih.gov/pmc/articles/PMC6043637.

5   Almeida, C. M. O. de and Malheiro, A. (2016). *Sleep, immunity and shift workers: A Review.* Sleep science (Sao Paulo, Brazil). Retrieved from https://www.ncbi.nlm.nih.gov/pmc/articles/PMC5241621.

6   Huang, S.-H.; Liao, C.-L.; Chen, S.-J.; Shi, L.-G.; Lin, L.; Chen, Y.-W.; Cheng, C.-P.; Sytwu, H.-K.; Shang, S.-T.; Lin, G.-J. (2019, May 7). *Melatonin possesses an anti-influenza potential through its immune modulatory effect.* Journal of Functional Foods. Retrieved from https://www.sciencedirect.com/science/article/pii/S1756464619302452.

7   Krueger, J. M. and Opp, M. R. (2016). *Sleep and microbes.* International review of neurobiology. Retrieved from https://www.ncbi.nlm.nih.gov/pmc/articles/PMC5441385.

8   Palma, B. D., search for more papers by this author; Gabriel Jr., A.; Colugnati, F. A. B.; Tufik, S. Address for reprint requests and other correspondence: B. D. Palma; Besedovsky, L.; & Zager, A. (2006, Nov. 1). *Effects of sleep deprivation on the development of autoimmune disease in an experimental model of systemic lupus erythematosus.* American Journal of Physiology-Regulatory, Integrative and Comparative Physiology. Retrieved from https://journals.physiology.org/doi/full/10.1152/ajpregu.00186.2006?url_ver=Z39.88-2003&rfr_id=ori%3Arid%3Acrossref.org&rfr_dat=cr_pub%3Dpubmed&.

9   Vaccaro, A.; Dor, Y.; Nambara , K. (2020, June 11). *Sleep Loss Can Cause Death through Accumulation of Reactive Oxygen Species in the Gut.* Cell. Retrieved from https://www.cell.com/cell/fulltext/S0092-8674(20)30555-9?_returnURL=https%3A%2F%2Flinkinghub.elsevier.com%2Fretrieve%2Fpii%2FS0092867420305559%3Fshowall%3Dtrue.

10   Walker, M. (2018). *Why we sleep: The new science of sleep and dreams.* Penguin.

11   Bierma, P. (2021, May 4). *Shift workers.* HealthDay. Retrieved from https://consumer.healthday.com/encyclopedia/work-and-health-41/occupational-health-news-507/shift-workers-646677.html.

12   Al;, P. J. J. L. B. J. H. (n.d.). *Differential effects of permanent and rotating shifts on self-report sleep length: A Meta-Analytic Review.* Sleep. Retrieved from https://pubmed.ncbi.nlm.nih.gov/10737332.

13   Magrini, A.; Pietroiusti, A.; Coppeta, L.; Babbucci, A.; Barnaba, E.; Papadia, C.; Iannaccone, U.; Boscolo, P.; Bergamaschi, E.; Bergamaschi, A. (n.d.). *Shift work and autoimmune thyroid disorders. International journal of immunopathology and pharmacology.* Retrieved from https://pubmed.ncbi.nlm.nih.gov/17291404.

14   Hedström, A. K.; Åkerstedt, T.; Klareskog, L.; Alfredsson, L. (2017, Aug. 1). *Relationship between shift work and the onset of rheumatoid arthritis.* RMD Open. Retrieved from https://rmdopen.bmj.com/content/3/2/e000475.

15   Costa, G. (2010, Dec.). *Shift work and Health: Current Problems and preventive actions.* Safety and health at work. Retrieved from https://www.ncbi.nlm.nih.gov/pmc/articles/PMC3430894.

16   Muir, H. (2001, May 21). *Air heads.* New Scientist. Retrieved from https://www.newscientist.com/article/dn765-air-heads/v.

17   *Researchers model unihemispheric sleep in humans.* Phys.org. (n.d.). Retrieved from https://phys.org/news/2019-07-unihemispheric-humans.html.

18   Banks, S., and Dinges, D. F. (2007, Aug. 15). *Behavioral and physiological consequences of sleep restriction.* Journal of clinical sleep medicine : JCSM : official publication of the American Academy of Sleep Medicine. Retrieved from https://www.ncbi.nlm.nih.gov/pmc/articles/PMC1978335.

19   *Blue Light has a dark side.* Harvard Health. (2020, July 7). Retrieved from https://www.health.harvard.edu/staying-healthy/blue-light-has-a-dark-side.

20   Wood, B.; Rea, M. S.; Plitnick, B.; Figueiro, M. G. (2012, July 31). *Light level and duration of exposure determine the impact of self-luminous tablets on melatonin suppression.* Applied Ergonomics. Retrieved from https://www.sciencedirect.com/science/article/abs/pii/S0003687012001159.

21   *Selected research articles, as of September, 2016 alpha . . .* (n.d.). Retrieved from https://alphastimforanimals.com/wp-content/uploads/2017/07/A-S_Website_-_Selected_Research_Articles_Sept__2016.pdf.

22 N;, H. A. B. (n.d.). *Use of ball blanket in attention-deficit/hyperactivity disorder sleeping problems.* Nordic journal of psychiatry. Retrieved from https://pubmed.ncbi.nlm.nih.gov/20662681.

23 Lastella, M.; O'Mullan, C.; Paterson, J. L.; Reynolds, A. C. (2019, March 4). *Sex and sleep: Perceptions of sex as a sleep promoting behavior in the general adult population.* Frontiers in public health. Retrieved from https://www.ncbi.nlm.nih.gov/pmc/articles/PMC6409294.

24 HP;, U. E. L. *Adenosine, caffeine, and performance: From cognitive neuroscience of sleep to sleep pharmacogenetics.* Current topics in behavioral neurosciences. Retrieved from https://pubmed.ncbi.nlm.nih.gov/24549722.

25 Institute of Medicine (US) Committee on Military Nutrition Research. (1970, Jan. 1). *Pharmacology of caffeine.* Caffeine for the Sustainment of Mental Task Performance: Formulations for Military Operations. Retrieved from https://www.ncbi.nlm.nih.gov/books/NBK223808.

26 L;, M. H. N. C. L. L. V. G. *Melatonin receptors in pancreatic islets: Good morning to a novel type 2 diabetes gene.* Diabetologia. Retrieved from https://pubmed.ncbi.nlm.nih.gov/19377888.

CHAPTER 7

Fasting

*F*ASTING HAS BEEN AROUND for thousands of years as a therapy for healing from illness. From the ancient Greeks, to Native Americans, to all the world's major religions, this obscure practice was developed independently from one group to another. Hippocrates, the father of Western medicine, believed fasting enabled the body to heal itself. Five hundred years ago, Paracelsus, another great healer in the Western tradition, wrote: "Fasting is the greatest remedy, the physician within."[1] Ayurvedic medicine has also long advocated fasting as a major treatment.

Benjamin Franklin (1706–1790), one of America's founding fathers and renowned for his wide knowledge in many areas, once wrote, "The best of all medicines is resting and fasting."[2] The ancient Greeks believed that medical treatments could be observed from nature, and humans, like most animals, naturally avoid eating when they become sick.

My only experiences with fasting up until my early 20s had been the Jewish holiday of Yom Kippur and trying to make weight for wrestling. The purpose of losing weight for wrestling was to dehydrate the body through shedding off water weight in order to make your weight class. This way, when you rehydrate after the weigh-in, you have a size advantage on your opponent. Looking back, I have no idea how I made it through those three-and-a-half-hour grueling practices on very little food and water, day in and day out. Our coach named a BAGUBA (Brutally Aggressive Guy Uninhibited By Adversity) at the end of each tournament or dual meet to honor the person who showed the most heart in their match, win or lose. As you begin your autoimmune journey, you must be a BAGUBA day in and day out and continually remind yourself of the HEALTH you want and deserve. And when it gets tough, perhaps during a fast, think or say aloud, "I feel super, I feel great," as we did during the thousands of repetitions of brutal physical combat.

The most basic form of fasting is intermittent fasting. Intermittent fasting or time-restricted eating are used interchangeably. They are defined by the daily transient fast lasting a minimum of 12 hours. For example, having your last meal at 8:00 p.m. and not eating again until 8:00 a.m. The fasting window can be increased to 14, 16, 18, or 24 hours. Time-restricted eating aligns with the body's natural circadian rhythm. We didn't always live in a time with access to 24-hour take-out. I had always bought into the myth that eating smaller meals throughout the day revved up the metabolism. I ate first thing in the morning and right before bed and all day in between. This myth has been disproved.

Some individuals already fast 12 hours as their normal routine. However, it was a bit of a lifestyle shift for me. As I adapted to that I began to incorporate 14- and then 16-hour fasts on most days, which included 2–3 meals during the feed window.

What exactly happens during the feasting window versus the fasting window? There exists a metabolic biochemical pathway, which has been named the mechanistic target of rapamycin or mTOR pathway. The mTOR pathway is responsible for anabolic muscle growth, which may be the goal for many bodybuilders and athletes looking to put on mass. This pathway is also infamously known for accelerating the aging process, when turned on chronically. Your activated protein kinase pathway, or AMPK, which is your body's main catabolic pathway, mobilizes your body's fuel sources while in a caloric deficit. During this time, a process known as cellular autophagy takes place, which literally means self-eating. This is your body's time to recycle any cells it has recognized as dysfunctional. This biochemical pathway is billions of years old and exists in bacteria. When food is absent, cells stop growing, and the aging process is halted.

There needs to be a balance between mTOR and AMPK; the dominance of mTOR, however, seems to be playing a large role in the manifestation of autoimmune disease and cancer. Rapamycin, a drug that is effective as an autophagy activator with mTOR inhibitory affects and led to a decrease of disease activity in a small group of Lupus patients.[3] In active Celiac disease, mTOR is over activated in the gut epithelium, which leads to the overreaction, growth, and proliferation of T cells.[4] As we age, autophagy activity decreases and contributes to the aging process.

Increased levels of glucose, insulin, and proteins all turn off autophagy. It doesn't take much. Even as little as 3 grams of the amino acid leucine can stop autophagy. The mTOR pathway is an important sensor of nutrient availability: When we eat carbohydrates or protein, insulin is secreted, and the increased insulin levels, or even just the amino acids from the breakdown of ingested protein, activate the mTOR pathway. The body senses that food is available and decides that, since there's plenty of energy to go around, there's no need to eliminate or recycle the old machinery. The end result is the suppression of autophagy. In other words, the constant intake of food, such as snacking throughout the day, suppresses autophagy. Conversely, when mTOR is dormant—when it's not being triggered by increased insulin levels or amino acids from ingested food—autophagy is promoted. As the body senses the temporary absence of nutrients, it must prioritize which cellular parts to keep. The oldest and most worn-out cellular parts get discarded, and amino acids from the broken-down cell parts are delivered to the liver, which uses them to create glucose during gluconeogenesis. It is not an all-

or-none principle because mTOR and AMPK pathways work proportionally.

It is likely that in the hunter-gatherer world, we went through periods of time with limited food and more commonly only ate 2–3 times a day. Autophagy promotes a controlled process of cellular recycling, preventing cells from becoming too old or dysfunctional. Conceptually, regular cycles of autophagy can prevent diseases such as cancer, neurodegeneration, cardiomyopathy, Diabetes, liver disease, autoimmune diseases, and infections. Furthermore, after going through a period of autophagy, it is important to refeed with ample amounts of protein in order to use the new stem cells to rebuild quality young muscle and tissues.

So far, scientists have discovered 32 genes associated with cellular autophagy. One example is the ATG16L gene. The inhibition or absence of this gene prevents autophagy of Paneth cells in the small intestine, which is responsible for the production of anti-microbial peptides. So, when the cells begin to become old and dysfunctional, the body is unable to break them down in order to create new ones, thus birthing gut inflammation. However, fasting turns genes off and on and mobilizes the production of stem cells, which are immature cells that can turn into whatever the body needs. The body can discriminate which cells or even organelles it chooses to break down, and yes, the hyperactive white blood cells of the immune system that cause autoimmunity are consumed first.[5] It has even been reported anecdotally that during prolonged fasts skin tags can be completely digested. Aside from your own cells, it also increases the breakdown of pathogenic bacteria. There are potential ways to increase autophagy during fasts through supplementation. However, for the purpose of this fast we want to focus on eliminating anything that might be triggering.

Exercise is widely recognized for its many health benefits, including lifespan expansion and protection against cardiovascular diseases, Diabetes, cancer, and neurodegenerative diseases. Studies that have been performed in mice show that exercise induces autophagy in the brain and several organs involved in metabolism, including the liver, pancreas, adipose tissue, and muscles, which may explain how exercise benefits the whole human body.[6]

Intermittent fasting and prolonged fasting have similar but different depths of effects. Intermittent fasting has been shown to decrease inflammation,[7] CRP, and cytokines.[8] Intermittent fasting leads to increased gut bacteria richness, enrichment of the good bacteria families, and enhanced antioxidative microbial metabolic pathways. Intermittent fasting alters T cells in the gut with a reduction of IL-17 producing T cells and an increase in regulatory T cells.[9]

Similarly to exercise, cold exposure, or certain toxins, intermittent fasting is an acute stressor. Acute stress on our body provides a beneficial hormetic response. This process is better known as hormesis. Hormesis is the concept of what doesn't kill you makes you stronger. Our body reacts to acute stressors by producing potent antioxidants, such as glutathione and superoxide dismutase, from the liver and releasing different protective hormones. When a stressor becomes chronic is when it can have deleterious long-term effects on our biologic systems by damaging our mitochondria. Chronic oxidative stressors can include overtraining, poor dietary choices, leaky gut syndrome, sleep deprivation, and starvation. On the other side of the token, carefully planned periodized fasting and short intense bouts of exercise can have a positive effect on health and longevity. However, someone who is overstressed should stick with the shorter intermittent fasts, to not overload their stress bank. During prolonged fasts it may be important to eliminate some of your controllable stress load such as decreasing the intensity and length of exercise, sauna, cold shower, etc.

Similar to the liver-producing antioxidants, in times of stress, the brain also becomes stressed! Whilst fasting, your body senses this stress and releases Brain-Derived Neurotrophic Factor (BDNF). BDNF's physiologic role is activating brain stem cells to convert into new neurons and thus promoting general neuronal health. This is effective in fighting age-related brain diseases. The combination of an intermittent fast and exercise play excellent synergy in the release of this robust peptide charged with protecting your noggin!

Another benefit of intermittent fasting is the huge increase in human growth hormone (HGH). HGH levels precipitously drop during aging. Normally HGH is secreted from the pituitary gland infrequently during the 24-hour circadian rhythm. Most of the HGH is secreted during deep sleep cycles; however, in fasting subjects, there was a significant increase in the pulsatile rate of HGH secretions as well as the amplitude of the secretions throughout the day. This means not only an increase in the number of times HGH is secreted, but also a greater volume of HGH secreted in each release. Perhaps the archaic reasoning for this phenomenon is to keep your body's substrate levels at homeostasis during periods of starvation. There is a plethora of studies ranging from intermittent fasts to one-day- to multiple-day-fasts—all resulting in robust increases in HGH. Cardiologists at the Intermountain Medical Center found that a 24-hour fast increased HGH by 1300 percent in women and almost 2000 percent in men.[10] HGH is one of the most important longevity hormones. When in a fasted state, HGH does not promote an increase in IGF-1, which is often a concern for cancer patients.

What is the best time for your feed window? Ideally earlier in the day. You don't have to eat right after rising, but you should leave several hours between your last meal and bed.

There exists a system in the brain called the glymphatic system. Its purpose is to filter out waste products in the brain similar to lymph fluid throughout the body. While you are asleep, the glymphatic system becomes 10 times more active than when you are awake, and your brain cells are reduced in size by 60 percent. The glymph clean-out requires a great amount of blood flow demand. Eating too soon before bed will shuttle blood to the digestive organs, inhibiting the ability to clean out the glymph in the brain. This illuminates the importance of leaving several hours before your last meal and bedtime. Dr. Steven Gundry, in *The Longevity Paradox*, recommends that you eat your last meal 4 hours before bed.[11] Preventing toxins from building up in your brain will increase the efficiency of your nervous system and endocrine system so you can continue to produce the most effective messages to the cells of your body.

Initially, start slow with the intermittent fast; stick to only 12 hours of fasting. Then you can work up to 16–18 hours and customize it to the way you feel. Some individuals do much better with the shorter intermittent fasts. Eventually, it will become so habitual you will think it was weird that you ever ate outside your fasting window.

Prolonged Fasts / Fasting Mimicking Diet

I never knew humans could go days without food and could sort of still thrive. It was a huge mental barrier I finally broke down. About a year after I began intermittent fasting, I began dabbling with more frequent 24-hour fasts. The first 36-hour fast I did really expanded what I thought humans were capable of. From there, 48 hours, 3 days, 5 days, and my longest fast to date has been 7 days.

The fasts are not a cake walk, and you will have your sticking points, but it's important to have a plan for when you get the fatigue or hunger pangs. This is no different than preparing for a triathlon. If you don't prepare and work up to it, you'll do pretty badly.

The longest therapeutic recorded fast was 382 days. This was an extreme case as the patient was over 456 pounds. Yes, humans can survive a weird amount of time without food so long as they have adequate calorie stores and supplement with micronutrients. However, we can only survive about 3 days without water.

For many with autoimmune disease, particularly in the gut, prolonged fasts may be of great importance in turning the tide of mTOR dominance, and allowing the gut to heal itself without any aggregating food triggers. Imagine if you keep brushing sandpaper across an open skin wound you have on your leg. You are preventing it from healing properly. This can be the case with an ulcered and leaky gut. The gut lining can turn over in just a few days, and fasting can give it the proper amount of time to heal.

One approach is the fasting mimicking diet (FMD) created by longevity researcher Dr. Valter Longo. It consists of a low-calorie fast over the course of 5 days. It's not quite as grueling as a 5-day fast, but you are in a steep calorie deficit, so you are still dipping into high levels of autophagy. The caloric range is around 500 calories. This approach is low in protein and high in plant carbohydrates, so it attempts to limit mTOR. My only caveat is that if you consume plants on this protocol that you are sensitive to, and trigger an immune response, it could defeat the whole purpose of doing the fast in the first place. However, the FMD is the most well-studied fasting protocol.

FMD can reduce white blood cell count by 40–50 percent during the fast. Then levels go back to normal when feeding resumes. However, due to the huge upregulation of stem cells, the new white blood cells are young and naïve. Each cycle of FMD decreases hyperactive white blood cells with fresh young ones.[12] FMD has been shown to regenerate insulin-producing cells of the pancreas in both Type I and Type II Diabetes.[13] In one version of the FMD, there were improvements in physical function, energy/fatigue, pain, and cognitive function in individuals with Multiple Sclerosis.[14] Rheumatoid Arthritis has also been shown to inhibit autophagy pathways. A 7–10 day FMD fast led to an improvement of the symptoms in many Rheumatoid Arthritis patients.[15]

In mice with IBD, FMD has been shown to be even more effective than water fasting alone, and it reduced intestinal inflammation, increased regenerative markers, promoted protective bacteria, and actually lengthened the size of the colon, thus showing regeneration.[16]

Ways to hack the fast

You must program your food cues. Various animals in labs have been trained to salivate when they see a white coat because they are fed shortly after. This conditions the animal to release certain hormones stimulating the digestive organs. This is the same reason that you shouldn't do anything in your bed but sleep. Cooking a meal or even just seeing and smelling food while fasting is almost unbearably difficult. This is not simply a matter of weak willpower. This, of course, is the same reason you should not shop for food when hungry or keep snacks in the pantry.

Before the fast you should condition yourself to eat only in the kitchen or at a certain table. Then, during the fast, you should avoid these environments as they will stimulate food cravings.

Tips for eating that can prepare you for a fast

- Eat only at the table
- Try to eat with another person/people
- No eating at your workstation
- No eating in the car
- No eating on the couch
- No eating in bed
- No eating while watching TV
- Try to avoid mindless eating—every meal should be enjoyed as a meal

Tips for curbing hunger during fast

- Brushing teeth or chewing gum can curb hunger
- Drink hot water, coffee, tea, bone broth
- Stay busy

The hunger will come in waves. Think back to a time when you skipped a meal. Perhaps you were caught up studying/working or not in your normal routine and couldn't get away. At first, you probably got "hangry." The hunger built and built, but your mind was on the task at hand and unable to tend to the hunger. However, after an hour or so the hunger disappeared. The wave had passed.

There are ways in which you can pass by the hunger phase as well. Drinking something hot like green tea, coffee, or water is often enough. Hunger does not continuously grow forever. It will build up, peak, and then disappear, and all you have to do is distract yourself from it. It will return, but remember it will pass again. Boredom is very dangerous while fasting and can cause you to crack. Try to stay busy as much as possible.

People can fast for days without feeling hungry. This is due to the fact that hunger is not determined by not eating for a certain period of time—hunger is a hormonal signal. It does not come about simply because the stomach is empty. When you avoid the hunger stimuli, such as the ones listed above, you can avoid the signal. Also, intermittent fasting and a whole foods diet will help you prepare by normalizing hormones: decreasing ghrelin levels (the hunger hormone) and increasing leptin (the satiation hormone). Studies on ghrelin show that with each consecutive day of a fast, peak ghrelin decreases.[17] The first 1–2 days of a fast are the hardest, and then it becomes significantly easier.

The best way to work up to an extended fast is by increasing the intermittent fast times or turning the body into ketosis. The keto diet usually consists of 70 percent fat, 20 percent protein, and 10 percent carbohydrates. The state of ketosis is when your liver runs out of stored glucose for energy so your body begins to break down stored fat. Fats are broken down into smaller molecules called ketone bodies that are then used for fuel. Training your body to use ketones for energy before a fast will better adapt you for the metabolic switch when your body runs out of stored glucose during the fast, thereby avoiding some of the side effects. This brings me to one of the benefits of prolonged fasting, which is a high level of circulating ketone bodies in the body. The most important ketone is Beta-hydroxybutyrate (BHB). BHB can feed the cells of your colon by crossing from the blood into the epithelium, thereby decreasing gut inflammation. This is especially important in individuals who don't have enough beneficial gut bacteria to produce butyrate for the cell wall. The ketogenic diet has also been shown to decrease pro-inflammatory T cells.[18]

Ketosis is the most important for neurological autoimmune diseases, including Epilepsy, seizures, Narcolepsy, Multiple Sclerosis,[19] Myasthenia Gravis, Guillain-Barre, or Encephalitis.[20] The protective effect for general seizures comes from the modulation of the gut microbiome.[21] Part of the benefit could also come from the fact that ketones are a much more efficient fuel for the brain and nervous system. For those with an overgrowth of bad bacteria that thrive on high fat, a keto diet may not be the way to go and can make symptoms worse.

Heart rate variability (HRV) is a measure of the difference in time between heartbeats. If your heart beats 60 times per minute, you would assume that means 1 beat per second. However, there is variability between heartbeats—in fact, the more variability, the greater the balance between the sympathetic and parasympathetic nervous system. In contrast, the lower the HRV, the more likely it is that one side of the nervous system is dominating, usually the sympathetic nervous system.[22] And, as previously explained, a dominant sympathetic response can tax the body. When I started consuming my last meal several hours before bed and during prolonged fasting, one of the first changes I noticed was the skyrocketing of my HRV. HRV can be measured with wearable devices such as the whoop band, aura ring, or fit bit. It is so important for autoimmune patients and those who are in remission to track HRV, because on days when you wake up and your HRV is low, that is your body's whisper to you to have a perfect couple of days of diet and recovery and to go light on the stress. If you are not adapted to fasting and you go into a prolonged fast, HRV may take a dive as that is too stressful on the body.

Who Should Not Fast

People who should not fast include those who are severely malnourished or underweight, children under age 18, pregnant or breastfeeding women, fragile individuals, those with liver or kidney disease, gout, someone who is taking medications that can interact with the fast, or if they have been prescribed iron supplementation.

There is no question about the benefits of intermittent fasting and prolonged fasting for the war on autoimmune disease, as long as the fasts are properly planned. This is one of the strategies that can really make a difference and should be implemented incrementally.

Happy Fasting!

NOTES

1   *Fasting – A history part I*. The Fasting Method. (2021, Aug. 31). Retrieved from https://blog.thefastingmethod.com/fasting-a-history-part-i.

2   *Fasting – A history part I*. The Fasting Method. (2021, Aug. 31). Retrieved from https://blog.thefastingmethod.com/fasting-a-history-part-i.

3   Fernandez, D. and Perl, A. (2010, March). *MTOR signaling: A central pathway to pathogenesis in systemic lupus erythematosus?* Discovery medicine. Retrieved from https://www.ncbi.nlm.nih.gov/pmc/articles/PMC3131182.

4   Sedda, S.; Dinallo, V.; Marafini, I.; Franzè, E.; Paoluzi, O. A.; Izzo, R.; Giuffrida, P.; Di Sabatino, A.; Corazza, G. R.; Monteleone, G. (2020, July 1). *MTOR sustains inflammatory response in celiac disease*. Nature News. Retrieved from https://www.nature.com/articles/s41598-020-67889-4.

5   Glick, D.; Barth, S.; Macleod, K. F. (2010, May). *Autophagy: Cellular and Molecular Mechanisms*. The Journal of Pathology. Retrieved from https://www.ncbi.nlm.nih.gov/pmc/articles/PMC2990190.

6   Escobar, K. A.; Cole, N. H.; Mermier, C. M.; VanDusseldorp, T. A. (2018, November 15). *Autophagy and aging: Maintaining the proteome through exercise and caloric restriction*. Wiley Online Library. Retrieved from https://onlinelibrary.wiley.com/doi/full/10.1111/acel.12876.

7   Vasconcelos, A. R.; Yshii, L. M.; Viel, T. A.; Buck, H. S.; Mattson, M.
     P.; Scavone, C.; Kawamoto, E. M. (2014, May 6). *Intermittent fasting
     attenuates lipopolysaccharide-induced neuroinflammation and memory
     impairment.* Journal of Neuroinflammation. Retrieved from https://link.
     springer.com/article/10.1186/1742-2094-11-85.

8   Aksungar, F. B.; Topkaya, A. E.; Akyildiz, M. (2007, March 19).
     *Interleukin-6, C-reactive protein and biochemical parameters during
     prolonged intermittent fasting.* Annals of Nutrition and Metabolism.
     Retrieved from https://www.karger.com/Article/PDF/100954.

9   Cignarella, F.; Cantoni, C.; Ghezzi, L.; Salter, A.; Dorsett, Y.; Chen, L.;
     Phillips, D.; Weinstock, G. M.; Fontana, L.; Cross, A. H.; Zhou, Y.; Piccio,
     L. (n.d.). *Intermittent fasting confers protection in CNS autoimmunity
     by altering the gut microbiota.* Cell metabolism. Retrieved from https://
     pubmed.ncbi.nlm.nih.gov/29874567.

10   ScienceDaily. (2011, May 20). *Routine periodic fasting is good for your
     health, and your heart, study suggests.* ScienceDaily. Retrieved from
     https://www.sciencedaily.com/releases/2011/04/110403090259.htm.

11   Gundry, S. R. and Lipper, J. (2019). *The longevity paradox: How to
     die young at a ripe old age.* Harper Luxe, an imprint of HarperCollins
     Publishers.

12   Choi, I. Y.; Piccio, L.; Childress, P.; Bollman, B.; Ghosh, A.; Brandhorst, S.;
     Suarez, J.; Michalsen, A.; Cross, A. H.; Morgan, T. E.; Wei, M.; Paul, F.;
     Bock, M.; Longo, V. D. (2016, June 7). *A diet mimicking fasting promotes
     regeneration and reduces autoimmunity and multiple sclerosis symptoms.*
     Cell reports. Retrieved from https://www.ncbi.nlm.nih.gov/pmc/articles
     /PMC4899145.

13   Cheng, C.-W.; Villani, V.; Buono, R.; Wei, M.; Kumar, S.; Yilmaz, O. H.;
     Cohen, P.; Sneddon, J. B.; Perin, L.; Longo, V. D. (2017, Feb. 23). *Fasting-
     mimicking diet promotes ngn3-driven β-cell regeneration to reverse
     diabetes.* Cell. Retrieved from https://www.ncbi.nlm.nih.gov/pmc/articles
     /PMC5357144.

14   Choi, I. Y.; Piccio, L.; Childress, P.; Bollman, B.; Ghosh, A.; Brandhorst,
     S.; Suarez, J.; Michalsen, A.; Cross, A. H.; Morgan, T. E.; Wei, M.; Paul,
     F.; Bock, M.; Longo, V. D. (2016, May 26). *A diet mimicking fasting
     promotes regeneration and reduces autoimmunity and multiple sclerosis
     symptoms.* Cell Reports. Retrieved from https://www.sciencedirect.com
     /science/article/pii/S2211124716305769.

15   *Effectiveness of therapeutic fasting and specific diet in patients with
     rheumatoid arthritis—full text view.* Effectiveness of Therapeutic Fasting
     and Specific Diet in Patients With Rheumatoid Arthritis - Full Text View
     - ClinicalTrials.gov. (n.d.). Retrieved from https://clinicaltrials.gov/ct2
     /show/NCT03856190.

16   Rangan, P.; Choi, I.; Wei, M.; Navarrete, G.; Guen, E.; Brandhorst, S.;
     Enyati, N.; Pasia, G.; Maesincee, D.; Ocon, V.; Abdulridha, M.; Longo,
     V. D. (2019, March 5). *Fasting-mimicking diet modulates microbiota and
     promotes intestinal regeneration to reduce inflammatory bowel disease*

pathology. Cell reports. Retrieved from https://www.ncbi.nlm.nih.gov/pmc/articles/PMC6528490.

17 Espelund, U.; Hansen, T. K.; Højlund, K.; Beck-Nielsen, H.; Clausen, J. T.; Hansen, B. S.; Orskov, H.; Jørgensen, J. O.; Frystyk, J. (n.d.). *Fasting unmasks a strong inverse association between ghrelin and cortisol in serum: Studies in obese and normal-weight subjects.* The Journal of clinical endocrinology and metabolism. Retrieved from https://pubmed.ncbi.nlm.nih.gov/15522942.

18 Ang, Q. Y.; Alexander, M.; Newman, J. C.; Tian, Y.; Cai, J.; Upadhyay, V.; Turnbaugh, J. A.; Verdin, E.; Hall, K. D.; Leibel, R. L.; Ravussin, E.; Rosenbaum, M.; Patterson, A. D.; Turnbaugh, P. J. (n.d.). *Ketogenic diets alter the gut microbiome resulting in decreased intestinal th17 cells.* Cell. Retrieved from https://pubmed.ncbi.nlm.nih.gov/32437658.

19 Storoni, M. and Plant, G. T. (2015, Dec. 29). *The therapeutic potential of the ketogenic diet in treating progressive multiple sclerosis.* Multiple Sclerosis International. Retrieved from https://www.hindawi.com/journals/msi/2015/681289.

20 McDonald, T. J. W. and Cervenka, M. C. (2018, Aug. 8). *The expanding role of ketogenic diets in adult neurological disorders.* Brain sciences. Retrieved from https://www.ncbi.nlm.nih.gov/pmc/articles/PMC6119973.

21 Olson, C. A.; Vuong, H. E.; Yano, J. M.; Liang, Q. Y.; Nusbaum, D. J.; Hsiao, E. Y. (n.d.). *The gut microbiota mediates the anti-seizure effects of the ketogenic diet.* Cell. Retrieved from https://pubmed.ncbi.nlm.nih.gov/29804833.

22 Marcelo Campos, M. D. (2019, Oct. 22). *Heart rate variability: A new way to track well-being.* Harvard Health. Retrieved from https://www.health.harvard.edu/blog/heart-rate-variability-new-way-track-well-2017112212789.

CHAPTER 8

Environmental Toxins

*E*VERY SECOND, OVER 680 POUNDS of toxic chemicals are released into our environment all around the world. Approximately 10 million tons of toxic chemicals are released into our environment each year. Of these, over 2 million tons per year are recognized carcinogens.[1] Our environment is getting more and more contaminated by chemicals, heavy metals, and dirty electricity.

It is fair to say that we are exposed to much higher levels of toxins than we would have been exposed to 15,000 years ago. In the realm of evolution, these are much greater levels of toxins than we evolved to detoxify. There are toxins in our air, in our products, in our food, and emanating from our technology. In fact, there are 212 chemicals found in the average person's blood or urine.[2]

There are three ways to deal with these artificially elevated levels of toxins: minimize the exposure to toxins, increase our body's resilience to stress, and increase the body's detoxification abilities. The toxic load from our environment is undoubtedly playing a role in the rising rates of autoimmune disease and contributes a fair share to the stress bank.

The body's detoxification mainly occurs in the liver in two phases. The toxins are transported to the liver via a fat-soluble compound. Then Phase I liver detox takes place, which includes converting toxins into metabolites, which actually makes the toxins more active and harmful. In Phase II liver detox, the toxins are manipulated in a way that allows them to be escorted out of the body. If detoxification pathways are not working properly, toxins can build up rapidly, and if Phase II liver detox is incapacitated, it could lead to some very harmful effects on the body. Some individuals who especially need to be careful are those with an inefficient gene variant of the MTHFR gene responsible for detoxification pathways. I am one of those individuals. It then becomes very important to seek higher levels of micronutrients that play a role in detoxification.

Phase 1 liver support includes nutrients: B vitamins; flavonoids; vitamins A, C, and E; glutathione; phospholipids; and various amino acids. (Grapefruit can decrease Phase 1, which is why it is a common contraindicator to drugs.)

Phase 2 support includes: Indole-3-carbonol (found in brassica vegetables), limonene (found in citrus fruits and some seeds), glutathione, fish oil, various amino acids, and NAC (N-acetyl cysteine).[3]

Detoxification gets complicated, and if done the wrong way it can make symptoms worse, which is why it is important to work closely with a health professional. Blood tests or urine tests can expose micronutrient deficiencies and environmental toxins that are contributing to excess toxic loads on the body. This approach can be used to strategically supplement and chelate toxins in order to rev up detoxification, while lowering harmful exposure.

The body has multiple other organ systems responsible for toxin removal. Some heavy metals as well as BPA can leave the body through the skin when we perspire.[4] The adrenal and thyroid glands are responsible for efficient function of the metabolism, and if these hormonal systems are hindered, a wrench will be thrown into the detoxification process. The kidneys, bladder, and bowels are the route for the elimination of toxins from the body.

In the gut, a healthy ecosystem of bacteria is the only way to efficiently eliminate the toxins in a non-leaky gut. For example, constipation will hamper the detoxification process and can lead to reabsorption of toxins into the bloodstream. The kidneys are responsible for filtering blood and producing urine, which is 95 percent water, and which is then passed out of the body. Therefore, many of the toxins need to be filtered through the kidneys. Drinking enough water is vital for efficient detoxification.

The lymphatic system is a network of vessels throughout the body that helps filter out the bad stuff. The vessels are connected by hubs called lymph nodes. When the body is overloaded by toxins or infections, lymph nodes tend to swell up. Increasing the filtration of the lymphatic system bolsters the immune system and helps detoxify the body.[5]

Heavy Metals

Heavy metals are naturally occurring elements that have usage in industrial, domestic, agricultural, medical, and technological industries, which has led to their heavy leakage into the environment. The toxicity to an exposed individual depends on different factors, including the dosage amount and route of exposure, as well as the person's age, gender, genetics, and nutritional status.

The most concerning heavy metals are arsenic, cadmium, chromium, lead, and mercury. These metallic elements are highly reactive in the body and are known to cause organ damage, even at lower levels of exposure. Heavy metals can adversely affect cellular organelles such as the cell membrane, mitochondria, lysosomes, and enzymes involved in metabolism, detoxification, and damage repair.[6] Other metals are actually needed by humans in small amounts for various biochemical and physiological functions. These include cobalt, copper, chromium, iron, magnesium, manganese, molybdenum, nickel, selenium, and zinc.

Where metals are found

Arsenic	Tap water, brown rice, herbicides, insecticides, wood preservatives, automobile exhaust, paint, cigarettes, fungicides, algicides, wood preservatives, and dyestuffs.
Aluminum	Tap water, antiperspirants, stomach antacids, household pots and pan, toothpaste, dental amalgams, cigarette filters, and tobacco smoke. For cooking, use parchment paper instead of aluminum foil and replace Teflon pans with stainless steel or enameled cast iron.
Cadmium	Cigarette smoke, tap water, paint pigments, fertilizers, alloys, and batteries.
Lead	Leaded gasoline fumes, paint, batteries, canned food with lead seams, meat and milk from animals that have been fed lead-contaminated food and can store it in their bones.
Nickel	Fertilizers, aerosols, and industrial dust.
Tin	Coated food cans, processed foods, industrial waste, and air pollution.
Mercury	Fish, amalgam fillings, mascara, contact lens solution, fabric softeners, vaccines, batteries with mercury cells, fungicides, and tap water.[7, 8]

Tips for eliminating your toxic environment

- Get all-natural fabrics for your bed, curtains, and carpets.

- Use natural hardwoods or bamboo for paneling.

- Use natural cleaning products like vinegar, baking soda, or hydrogen peroxide for cleaning. A lot of popular cleansing brands have high levels of toxic chemicals such as 1,4-Dioxane, DEA, and TEA.

- Get rid of the toxic artificial air fresheners and switch to natural essential oils. However, there are a select few essential oils that have hormonal effects when absorbed through the skin.

- Paint with low-volatile organic compounds indoors.

In dentistry, amalgams used to contain mercury that has been measured to leak. The World Health Organization states that mercury amalgams are safe, although side effects can occur.[9] Longitudinal studies point that over the long haul there was no increase in neurologic symptoms.[10] However, these are correlative studies and are not able to control for thousands of confounding factors. In an immune-compromised individual, it isn't one toxin that is the problem, but rather the compounded effect of them together. Therefore, it is important to limit the net toxic load. Some individuals may have a hypersensitivity to mercury, and for them the consequences can be more severe.

If you are concerned about the toxic load on your body and if you have high mercury levels, there is a nontoxic alternative to amalgam called a composite filling, or "white filling." They are readily available and offered by many dentists. If you need a dental filling, ask your dentist to do a composite. One reason we are so concerned about amalgam fillings today is that they were the only type of filling offered for many decades, thus most people have them. They are also less expensive than composites, which makes them more attractive. There is much concern about mercury leaking in the mouth and then into the rest of the body.

Another important note is just because a fish is wild does not mean it does not have high levels of mercury. Mercury was one of the toxins that was very high in my body, and I had very high amounts of mercury antibodies, telling me it was contributing to chronic low grade inflammation. It is best to avoid bigger fish such as tuna, sharks, and swordfish.

Hygiene / Cosmetic Products

Within seconds of applying shampoos or lotions, pseudo estrogens can be absorbed into the body and disrupt the endocrine system. The skin is the largest organ of the body and has a significant amount of surface area to absorb chemicals. It is important to look at the labels on shampoos, soaps, sunscreens, conditioners, toothpaste, deodorants, and others. The artificial ingredients in some of the products can be hypersensitive to some individuals and cause an immune reaction. Some of the common plastic chemicals are BPA, phthalates, triclosan, and PCBs, all of which have estrogenic effects with the body. This can partially explain earlier puberty in females in Western society and reduced sperm count in males. UV light, microwaves, and heat cause the bleaching of harmful compounds in plastics.[11] Babies who are given medical plastic tubing for oxygen can have circulating plastics in the blood that are up to 4000–160,000 times higher than safe levels.[12]

Water

Filtering water is very important in order to remove industrial toxins. Reverse Osmosis (RO) is the best water treatment process because it removes many of the harmful pollutants that other filters cannot. RO eliminates pharmaceuticals, chlorine, fluoride, pesticides, sulfates, nitrates, and heavy metals. Chlorine is put into the water for its antimicrobial properties, but even low levels can alter the microbiome.[13] You can find RO water refill stations at many supermarkets and fill up mason jars for about 30 cents a gallon. If you have access to natural spring water from a clean source, this may be one of the best ways to consume water because its mineral content ordinarily gets filtered out during the filtration process. Some individuals fortify their filtered water with minerals to make up for this deficiency.

Toothpaste

Swallowing too much toothpaste can be fatal. We don't very often have warnings like that for stuff we put in our mouths. Yes, toothpaste has the ability to fight off tooth decay, but if you are respecting your body with the right foods and ample amounts of fat-soluble vitamins, tooth decay is nothing to worry about. The heavy levels of artificial ingredients and high amounts fluoride are not something our ancestors were exposed to through products or food, and we know from anthropological research of tribes and communities on ancestral diets that tooth decay was almost nonexistent.[14]

In areas of the country where fluoride fortification in the drinking water supply is in the upper limits and individuals are stacking it with fluoride-enhanced toothpaste, kids can easily go over what is deemed a safe level. There have been links to fluoride consumption and inhibited cognitive development, thyroid function, and brittle bones.[15] If you are following an ancestral diet, seek out an all-natural toothpaste without fluoride and avoid alcohol-based mouth wash that can nuke the oral microbiome. However, if you are not on an ancestral diet and do not consume enough fat-soluble vitamins, then it is important to use fluoride-fortified toothpaste to protect your teeth from self-inflicted decay.

Female Products

Female hygiene products such as tampons can contain BPA and other endocrine disruptors or synthetic materials. Even certain cotton products may contain heavy amounts of pesticides. Plastics could cause all sorts of fertility issues.

Water Bottles

Switch from disposable plastic water bottles over to a stainless-steel reusable water bottle or glass mason jars.

Cosmetic Products

Cosmetics can contain chemicals such as BHA, BHT, TEA, phthalates, or triclosan. Lipsticks, eyeliners, and other products are applied right next to open orifices so they can be ingested. Seek out safe products.

Molds / Mycotoxins

Molds are a type of fungi and produce a toxin called mycotoxins.

Molds can thrive in an environment with a lot of moisture and oxygen.

Mold can have a musty smell.

As explained in Chapter 4, mold is not just toxic to humans, but also to bacteria, which is why it is used in antibiotics.[16]

Ways to prevent mold overgrowth is to keep humidity down throughout your home, open the windows and allow for a free flow of air, and make sure there are no water leaks. Mold can grow in as little as 24–48 hours.

If you expect you might have a mold problem, a licensed contractor can provide you with an environmental relative moldiness index. This will determine how much toxic mold is in your house. You can also find out yourself with an at-home kit.

For the majority of people, their greatest source of mold is from food. Foods high in mycotoxin molds are corn products, wheat, peanuts, peanut butter, coffee, sour cream, lunch meats, salami, smoked fish, and leftovers in the refrigerator.

Air Quality

In the industrialized world, humans spend over 90 percent of their time in indoor spaces![17] Air pollution can impair T cell function, increase inflammation, and is linked to asthma.[18] It is important to open windows as much as possible to filter the air. Pollutants are much higher indoors, illuminating the importance of getting a fine air filter that can filter mold, dust, dander, and other toxins from the air. The HEPA air filter is one possible choice and is capable of removing particles as small as 0.1 microns. They use a technology developed by NASA called advanced hydration photocatalytic oxidation, or AHPCO, which destroys mold, bacteria, and other microorganisms with ultraviolet light and a catalyst. NASA also did research on pollution-reducing plants in living and workspaces: these can include bamboo palm, mums, English ivy, Chinese Evergreen, Aloe Vera, Snack plant, or Spider plant. These plants actually neutralize certain chemicals such as formaldehyde, benzene, and trichloroethylene from the air.[19]

Pesticides / GMO

Pesticides are found on many produce items. Eating organic foods or shopping at farmers' markets are great ways to avoid food chemicals. Getting organic certification can be really expensive, and often local farmers who sell at farmers markets are referred to as beyond organic. They follow even stricter practices than large organic farms, but they may not be certified as organic. Some fruits and vegetables are notorious for having much more pesticide residue than others. They are referred to as the dirty dozen and are non-negotiables for always purchasing organic: strawberries, spinach, kale, nectarines, apples, grapes, cherries, peaches, pears, peppers, celery, and tomatoes. It is important in today's world to wash all fruits and vegetables and keep in mind washing them does not get rid of all the pesticides. This is unfortunate because the microbes in the dirt which end up on produce have beneficial effects on our microbiome.

The most ubiquitous pesticide is glyphosate, created by the infamous Monsanto. In 2012, 290 million pounds were dumped onto crops.[20] Besides bathing our crops, the chemical finds its way into runoff and into our water. Glyphosate seems to have deleterious effects on our gut bacteria including acting as an endocrine disruptor, chelating minerals,[21] and ravaging the gut lining, thereby increasing the risk of Celiac disease.[22]

DDT (dichlorobiphenyl-trichloroethane) is a pesticide that was outlawed in the United States in the 1970s because it is potently toxic. However, it can still be found in soil and carpeting in people's homes. Studies show that pesticides are mostly brought into the home via shoes and can be brought up into the air for 30 minutes after sweeping.[23] Studies of farmers who use pesticides show a link toward increased prevalence of ANA antibodies and Systematic Autoimmune Disease.[24] Pesticides have endangered entire species. Take steps to remove shoes at the door of the house so you are not bringing in toxic residue.

Genetically Modified Crops

Genetically modified crops (GMOs) are designed by taking DNA from an animal or plant and putting it into crops for desired traits. There are bananas that produce human vaccines against infectious diseases such as hepatitis B, fish that glow in the dark, and fruit and plants that produce plastics with unique properties. Most commonly, genes are spliced in to increase plant toxins (enzyme inhibitors, saponins, or lectins) or to tolerate spray pesticides better. They can also be designed to increase mineral and vitamin content. Corn and soybeans are the most common GMOs in the United States. Knowing how damaging spray pesticides can be on the gut, I think it is generally safe to stay away from GMO pesticides during the healing phase from autoimmune disease.

Noise Pollution

According to the European environment agency, noise is responsible for 16,000 premature deaths a year and 72,000 hospitalizations.[25] Noise pollution can be defined as any noise above 65 dB, and it becomes damaging above 85 decibels. A car horn is around 90-100 dB.

Chronic noise exposure can be considered an environmental stress or toxin. Also, it upregulates cortisol production and therefore chronically can depress the immune system.[26] This can become a big problem for construction workers, military, and law enforcement, as well as for honking in cities and living near airports or trains.

Ways to prevent noise pollution

- Turn down the speakers and headphones.
- Avoid loud noisy places. Nightclubs and concerts may not be the best spot during the healing phase of autoimmune disease.
- If listening to loud music, take breaks.
- Use earplugs and headphones when you can't avoid loud sounds.
- At events, stay away from the loudest speakers.

EMFs

EMFs is short for electrical magnetic fields. They can vary in frequency and wave. EMFs can come from natural sources such as the sun or man-made sources like cell phones, Wi-Fi, microwaves, and wiring. In today's world we are exposed to one quintillion more EMFs than we were just 100 years ago.[27]

There are two types of EMFs: ionizing and nonionizing radiation.

- Ionizing EMFs have the power to disrupt an atom by knocking off one or more electrons, causing the atom to gain a positive charge. This causes free radicals in the human body. Ionizing radiation causes DNA damage, and in well known cases like overdosing on X-rays, it can result in serious health effects.

- Nonionizing radiation comes from electronics, smart devices, Wi-Fi, and Bluetooth. This type of radiation also produces free radicals and damage to your cells. In fact, cell phone manufacturers recommend you never hold the phone directly to your head.

EMFs use AC or alternating currents, unlike the DC or direct current that emits from the Earth and is used in our bodies. The unnatural EMFs are all almost impossible to escape from in the modern world, and our bodies react to them similarly to the way they react to other environmental stressors. Dirty electricity can most often range from 2,000–100,000 Hz. The mechanistic way in which EMFs are harmful is that when they interact with cell membranes they cause an abnormal amount of calcium to flood into the cell, resulting in cellular damage and decreasing ATP production.[28, 29] Dirty electricity can be found in fluorescent bulbs, solar panels, many LED lights, hair dryers, refrigerators, televisions, smart appliances, and cell towers. The lower the bar on your phone or the worse the connection, the more EMFs being produced. The cleanest connection is in your house. Cell phone service is dependent on towers that receive and transmit

EMFs/radiofrequencies, and in order to increase cell service and bandwidth, more cell towers are continuing to be built up with more powerful signaling. As we upgrade from 4G to 5G, the Hz power increases, and it is yet unknown what the consequences might be.

Avoid using your cell phone when the connection is bad. Phones emit up to 10,000 times more EMF radiation when connectivity is low.[30] Also, when making phone calls or if you're on the internet, the phone increases EMF production, more than when it is not being used for those functions. Use speaker phone or corded headphones when possible.

Similarly to how some individuals have hypersensitivities to certain foods or environmental molecules, there are individuals who have hypersensitivity to EMFs and are more heavily effected than others. In addition, EMFs have been shown to impact HRV[31] and alter bacteria growth.[32]

You cannot always control the environment outside your house. But within your walls it is important to make your home a sanctuary away from dirty electricity. If EMF exposure is something you are concerned about, building biologists— professionals who identify and eliminate chemical, mold, electric, magnetic, and radio-frequency irritants—can come to your residence. You can also purchase meters that are able to seek out the source of dirty electricity.

When grounded with the earth or a device, EMFs have less of a deleterious effect on the body and do not get rattled voltage potentials throughout the body.

For more information, Chapter 10 offers in-depth insight on what it means to be electrically grounded. Also, you can learn even more about the harmful effects of EMFs in the book *EMF*D* by Dr. Joe Mercola.

Vaccines

Other factors that can contribute to increased rates of autoimmunity are both viruses and vaccines. (See Chapter 4 for a history of modern viruses.) Vaccines contain toxic additives such as aluminum, mercury, formaldehyde, etc. These toxins are sometimes added as preservatives or in order to maximize an immune response to ensure that the vaccination provokes a strong enough response so the body remembers it for future exposure. Unluckily for those with autoimmunity, our immune systems are already over-activated, and this can tip the scale as documented with Guillain-Barre, Narcolepsy, and Thrombocytopenia.[33, 34, 35] With that being said, there is an even greater increase in autoimmune disease associated with infection from the virus that the vaccine seeks to preclude. On a population level there is no question that vaccines are an effective healthcare measure and save lives. However, strategically, a case can be made on the individual level that measures the risk of obtaining a virus with the insulin sensitivity, micronutrient status, and general health of the individual.

In the future there may be a more personalized approach to vaccination that takes into account genetics, body weight, or gender, thereby tailoring the dosage to the individual to prevent unwanted side effects. If you have a teeming autoimmune disease, I recommend monitoring how your body feels immediately, days, and weeks after a vaccine to see if it in fact contributes to your disease. Speak to your doctor before receiving vaccines, because in certain individuals with autoimmune disease there are clear contraindications. Whether the benefits outweigh the costs to your health is case by case and depends on the of type of vaccine and disease you are trying to prevent.

Examples of ubiquitous toxins

Dichlorobenzene	Found in disinfectants, deodorants, insecticides, metal polishes, and paints.[36]
Xylene	Found in printing products, rubber paint, ink, cigarette smoke, plastics, insecticides, and petroleum products.[37]
Toluene	Found in, carpets, copy paper, paint, and petroleum products.[38]
Chloroform	Found in cleaning solvents, artificial silk, floor polishes, and insecticides.[39]
Trichloroethylene (TCE)	Found in dry-cleaning products, metal degreasers, and stain removers. TCE is also used in printing inks, varnishes, adhesives, and paints.[40]
Hexane/heptane/ pentanes	Found in glue, cement, adhesives, paint thinner, plastics, gasoline, and ink.[41]
Formaldehyde	Found in foam insulation, pressed wood products, backing on carpet, cigarette smoke, grocery bags, facial tissues, paper towels, and vaccines.[42]
Benzene	Found in cigarette smoke, rubber, secondhand smoke, gasoline, pesticides, oils, plastics, detergents, pharmaceuticals, paints, and dyes.[43]

BPA	Identified in most bags that hold common processed foods like chips or cookies, ice cube trays, shampoo bottles, frozen food containers, straws, Tupperware, takeout containers, and plastic utensils. Even BPA-free products are not desirable, because they use other plastics that have not been studied and may take many years to expose potential harm.
	Ditch the plastic Tupperware and the disposable water bottles and switch to glass or stainless steel.[44]

Treating Toxic Overload

Chelation Therapy uses various binders that are each injected via IV or swallowed as a pill in order to bind to heavy metals and bring them out of the body. The human body produces some chelators naturally like NAC, lipoic acid, glutathione, N-acetylcysteine, and cysteine. Medical chelation has been shown in animal studies and case reports to decrease symptoms associated with autoimmune disease.[45] Chelation has multiple benefits aside from eliminating toxins; it also reduces free-radical activity and improves blood flow.

Anyone with autoimmunity who has heavy metal toxicity must have the heavy metals neutralized in order to heal, and chelation is the most effective way to achieve this. Several herbal and nutritional approaches, although less effective, can be used by people who do not wish to undergo medical chelation

Sauna therapy, dry skin brushing, and rebounding are all-natural therapies that can help detoxify the body. See Chapter 10 for more on these therapies.

A Look at the Chelators

There may be some side effects to chelation therapy.

Individuals with mild or moderate kidney problems should be monitored closely during treatment to avoid overloading the kidneys. Due to the role of chelators binding to toxins in the body and guiding them out, micronutrients may also be removed in the process. Depending on which chelator is used, micronutrient supplementation may be necessary. There also can be other side effects associated with chelation such as fever, headache, nausea, diarrhea, and organ damage.

DMPS (2,3-dimercaptopropane-1-sulfonate) is a chelator used for the removal of mercury, lead, arsenic, cadmium, nickel, tin, and other metals. DMPS can be taken 3 different ways: orally, intravenously, or in suppository form.

DMSA (2,3-dimercaptosuccinic acid) is a chelator given to remove mercury, lead, and arsenic from the body. One feature that makes DMSA unique from DMPS is its ability to cross the blood-brain barrier, which means it can chelate heavy metals that have reached the brain.

EDTA (ethylene diamine tetraacetic acid) is a chelator used to remove metals such as aluminum, cadmium, lead, and tins.[46, 47, 48]

Herbal Chelators

Some herbal/food chelators that can be used as part of a detoxification and chelation protocol include: uva ursi (*Arctostaphylos uva-ursi*), burdock root (*Arctium lappa*), lemon balm (*Melissa officinalis*), spirulina, milk thistle (*Silybum marianum*), yellow dock (*Rumex crispus*), and dandelion root (*Taraxacum officinale*).

It is very clear that we live in a world where humans are exposed to chemicals and toxins at unnaturally high levels. We therefore must test for exposure and eliminate daily sources of harmful toxins. This means seeking clean food/water sources, eliminating excess radiation, and using clean products.

NOTES

1   *Toxic chemicals released by industries this year, tons.* Worldometer. (n.d.). Retrieved Nov. 3, 2021, from https://www.worldometers.info/view /toxchem.

2   *Fourth report in human Exposure to Environemental Chemicals.* (n.d.). Retrieved Nov. 3, 2021, from https://www.cdc.gov/exposurereport/pdf /FourthReport.pdf.

3   http://humanaalimentar.com.br/custom/308/uploads/profissional /Nutritional_Detoxifcation_clinical_Practice.pdf

4   Sears, M. E.; Kerr, K. J.; Bray, R. I. (2012). *Arsenic, cadmium, lead, and Mercury in sweat: A systematic review.* Journal of environmental and public health. Retrieved from https://www.ncbi.nlm.nih.gov/pmc/articles /PMC3312275.

5   Zimmermann, K. A. (2018, Feb. 21). *Lymphatic system: Facts, functions & diseases.* LiveScience. Retrieved from https://www.livescience.com/26983 -lymphatic-system.html.

6   Tchounwou, P. B.; Yedjou, C. G.; Patlolla, A. K.; Sutton, D. J. (2012). *Heavy metal toxicity and the environment.* Experientia supplementum (2012). Retrieved from https://www.ncbi.nlm.nih.gov/pmc/articles /PMC4144270.

7   *The main sources of heavy metals in the soil and pathways . . .* (n.d.). Retrieved from https://www.researchgate.net/publication/332543308_THE _MAIN_SOURCES_OF_HEAVY_METALS_IN_THE_SOIL_AND _PATHWAYS_INTAKE.

8   Klotz, K.; Weistenhöfer, W.; Neff, F.; Hartwig, A.; van Thriel, C.; Drexler, H. (2017, Sept. 29). *The health effects of aluminum exposure.* Deutsches Arzteblatt international. Retrieved from https://www.ncbi.nlm.nih.gov /pmc/articles/PMC5651828.

9   Mjör, I. A. and Pakhomov, G. N., eds. Dental amalgam and alternative direct restorative materials. World Health Organization Consultation on Assessing the Risks and Benefits to Health Oral Care and the Environment using Dental Amalgam and Its Replacement. 2007 March 3–7; Geneva. Geneva: World Health Organization; 1997, p xi.

10 DeRouen, T. A.; Martin, M. D.; Leroux, B. G.; Townes, B. D.; Woods, J. S.; Leitão, J.; Castro-Caldas, A.; Luis, H.; Bernardo, M.; Rosenbaum, G.; Martins, I. P. Neurobehavioral effects of dental amalgam in children: a randomized clinical trial. JAMA 2006;295:1784-1792.

11 Yang, C. Z.; Yaniger, S. I.; Jordan, V. C.; Klein, D. J.; Bittner, G. D. (2011, July). *Most plastic products release estrogenic chemicals: A potential health problem that can be solved.* Environmental health perspectives. Retrieved from https://www.ncbi.nlm.nih.gov/pmc/articles/PMC3222987.

12 MA;, M. E. B. F. (n.d.). *Phthalates and critically ill neonates: Device-related exposures and non-endocrine toxic risks.* Journal of perinatology : official journal of the California Perinatal Association. Retrieved from https://pubmed.ncbi.nlm.nih.gov/25357096.

13   *(PDF) the effects of chlorinated drinking water on the Assembly of the intestinal microbiome*. ResearchGate. (n.d.). Retrieved from https://www. researchgate.net/publication/330537336_The_Effects_of_Chlorinated _Drinking_Water_on_the_Assembly_of_the_Intestinal_Microbiome.

14   Nutri Price, W. (2010). *Nutrition and physical degeneration: A comparison of primitive and modern diets and their effects*. Garsington.

15   Peckham, S. and Awofeso, N. (2014, Feb. 26). *Water fluoridation: A critical review of the physiological effects of ingested fluoride as a public health intervention*. TheScientificWorldJournal. Retrieved from https://www.ncbi .nlm.nih.gov/pmc/articles/PMC3956646.

16   Bennett, J. W. and Klich, M. (2003, July). *Mycotoxins*. Clinical microbiology reviews. Retrieved from https://www.ncbi.nlm.nih.gov/pmc /articles/PMC164220.

17   Environmental Protection Agency. (n.d.). EPA. Retrieved from https:// www.epa.gov/indoor-air-quality-iaq/inside-story-guide-indoor-air-quality.

18   Bauer, R. N.; Diaz-Sanchez, D.; Jaspers, I. (2012, January). *Effects of air pollutants on innate immunity: The role of toll-like receptors and nucleotide-binding oligomerization domain-like receptors*. The Journal of allergy and clinical immunology. Retrieved, from https://www.ncbi.nlm .nih.gov/pmc/articles/PMC4341993.

19   *NASA reveals a list of the best air-cleaning plants for your home*. Bored Panda. Retrieved from https://www.boredpanda.com/best-air-filtering -houseplants-nasa/.

20   Environmental Protection Agency. (n.d.). EPA. Retrieved from https:// www.epa.gov/pesticides/pesticides-industry-sales-and-usage-2006-and -2007-market-estimates.

21   Myers, J. P.; Antoniou, M. N.; Blumberg, B.; Carroll, L.; Colborn, T.; Everett, L. G.; Hansen, M.; Landrigan, P. J.; Lanphear, B. P.; Mesnage, R.; Vandenberg, L. N.; Vom Saal, F. S.; Welshons, W. V.; Benbrook, C. M. (2016, February 17). *Concerns over use of glyphosate-based herbicides and risks associated with exposures: A consensus statement*. Environmental health : a global access science source. Retrieved from https://www.ncbi .nlm.nih.gov/pmc/articles/PMC4756530.

22   Samsel, A. and Seneff, S. (2013, December). *Glyphosate, pathways to modern diseases II: Celiac sprue and gluten intolerance*. Interdisciplinary toxicology. Retrieved from https://www.ncbi.nlm.nih.gov/pmc/articles /PMC3945755.

23   U.S. Department of Health and Human Services. (n.d.). *Distribution of pesticides and polycyclic aromatic hydrocarbons in house dust as a function of particle size*. National Institute of Environmental Health Sciences. Retrieved from https://ehp.niehs.nih.gov/doi/10.1289/ehp.99107721.

24   Parks, C. G.; Santos, A. de S. E.; Lerro, C. C.; DellaValle, C. T.; Ward, M. H.; Alavanja, M. C.; Berndt, S. I.; Beane Freeman, L. E.; Sandler, D. P.; Hofmann, J. N. (1AD, January 1). *Lifetime pesticide use and antinuclear antibodies in male farmers from the Agricultural Health Study*.

Frontiers. Retrieved from https://www.frontiersin.org/articles/10.3389/fimmu.2019.01476/full.

25 Corporativa, I. (n.d.). *Noise pollution: How to reduce the impact of an invisible threat?* Iberdrola. Retrieved from https://www.iberdrola.com/environment/what-is-noise-pollution-causes-effects-solutions.

26 Kim, A.; Sung, J. H.; Bang, J.-H.; Cho, S. W.; Lee, J.; Sim, C. S. (2017, October 30). *Effects of self-reported sensitivity and road-traffic noise levels on the immune system.* PloS one. Retrieved from https://www.ncbi.nlm.nih.gov/pmc/articles/PMC5662213.

27 Johansson, O. and Flydal, E. "Health Risk from Wireless? The debate is over" Electromagentichealth.org (blog). 2014.

28 Pall, M. L. "Wi-fi is an important threat to human health." environmental research. https://pubmed.ncbi.nlm.nih.gov/29573716.

29 Vekaria, H. J. "targeting mitochondrial dysfunction in CNS injury using methylene blue; still a magic bullet?" Neurochemical international. https://pubmed.ncbi.nlm.nih.gov/28396091.

30 Wall, S.; Wang, Z.-M.; Kendig, T.; Dobraca, D.; Lipsett, M. (2018, Oct. 3). *Real-world cell phone radiofrequency electromagnetic field exposures.* Environmental Research. Retrieved from https://www.sciencedirect.com/science/article/abs/pii/S0013935118305024?via%3Dihub.

31 VD;, P. I. L. A. G. N. E. L. D. O. (n.d.). *[the effect of low-intensity millimeter-range electromagnetic radiation on the cardiovascular system of the white rat].* Fiziologicheskii zhurnal SSSR imeni I. M. Sechenova. Retrieved from https://pubmed.ncbi.nlm.nih.gov/1330714.

32 A;, S. D. T. K. T. (n.d.). *Millimeter waves or extremely high frequency electromagnetic fields in the environment: What are their effects on bacteria?* Applied microbiology and biotechnology. Retrieved from https://pubmed.ncbi.nlm.nih.gov/27087527.

33 F;, H. P. S. J. M. Y. D. S. (n.d.). *Vaccines and Guillain-Barré syndrome.* Drug safety. Retrieved from https://pubmed.ncbi.nlm.nih.gov/19388722.

34 MM;, S. T. O. A. A. P. E. D. Y. A. P. (n.d.). *Incidence of narcolepsy after H1N1 influenza and vaccinations: Systematic review and meta-analysis.* Sleep medicine reviews. Retrieved from https://pubmed.ncbi.nlm.nih.gov/28847694.

35 Cecinati, V.; Principi, N.; Brescia, L.; Giordano, P.; Esposito, S. (2013, May). *Vaccine administration and the development of immune thrombocytopenic purpura in children.* Human vaccines & immunotherapeutics. Retrieved from https://www.ncbi.nlm.nih.gov/pmc/articles/PMC3899154.

36 *Dichlorobenzene) 1,4-dichlorobenzene (para- - epa.gov.* (n.d.). Retrieved from https://www.epa.gov/sites/default/files/2016-09/documents/1-4-dichlorobenzene.pdf.

37 Kandyala, R.; Raghavendra, S. P. C.; Rajasekharan, S. T. (2010, Jan.). *Xylene: An overview of its health hazards and preventive measures.* Journal of oral and maxillofacial pathology : JOMFP. Retrieved from https://www.ncbi.nlm.nih.gov/pmc/articles/PMC2996004.

38   *Department of Labor Logo United Statesdepartment of Labor.* Toluene—Overview | Occupational Safety and Health Administration. (n.d.). Retrieved from https://www.osha.gov/toluene.

39   *Chloroform—US EPA.* (n.d.). Retrieved from https://www.epa.gov/sites/production/files/2016-09/documents/chloroform.pdf.

40   *Trichloroethylene (TCE) and your health.* EH: Minnesota Department of Health. (n.d.). Retrieved from https://www.health.state.mn.us/communities/environment/hazardous/topics/tce.html.

41   *Comparative estimation of the neurotoxic risks . . . springer.* (n.d.). Retrieved from https://link.springer.com/chapter/10.1007/978-1-4757-9480-9_50.

42   *Formaldehyde.* American Cancer Society. (n.d.). Retrieved from https://www.cancer.org/cancer/cancer-causes/formaldehyde.html.

43   *Benzene and cancer risk.* American Cancer Society. (n.d.). Retrieved from https://www.cancer.org/cancer/cancer-causes/benzene.html.

44   *Fourth report in human Esposure to Environemental Chemicals.* (n.d.). Retrieved Nov. 3, 2021 from https://www.cdc.gov/exposurereport/pdf/FourthReport.pdf.

45   Rupress.org.   (n.d.).   Retrieved   from   https://rupress.org/jem/article/160/5/1532/23453/Inhibition-of-autoimmune-neuropathological-process.

46   Dans, A. L.; Tan, F. N.; Villarruz-Sulit, E. C. (2002, Oct. 21). *Chelation therapy for atherosclerotic cardiovascular disease - dans, al - 2002: Cochrane Library.* Cochrane Database of Systematic Reviews. Retrieved from   https://www.cochranelibrary.com/cdsr/doi/10.1002/14651858.CD002785/abstract.

47   Bamonti, F.; Fulgenzi, A.; Novembrino, C.; Ferrero, M. E. (2011, June 8). *Metal chelation therapy in Rheumathoid arthritis: A case report.* BioMetals. Retrieved from https://link.springer.com/article/10.1007%252Fs10534-011-9467-9.

48   Kannan, G. M. and Flora, S. J. S. (n.d.). *Combined administration of N-acetylcysteine and monoisoamyl DMSA on tissue oxidative stress during arsenic chelation therapy.* Biological Trace Element Research. Retrieved from https://link.springer.com/article/10.1385/BTER:110:1:43.

CHAPTER 9

Exercise

*F*ROM CROSSFIT TO POWERLIFTING, from bodybuilding to calisthenics, I have experimented with almost every facet of trendy fitness out there. Now I train to be pain free and to feel like a billion bucks. This chapter explains how important fitness is for autoimmune disease.

Only about 23 percent of Americans get the daily recommended dose of exercise.[1] We also spend most of our days seated. It is recommended to get 150 minutes of moderate exercise per week to lower risk for chronic disease. Even if you're getting 3–4 hours a week of exercise, if you are sitting for most of the rest of the time, there will still be a high risk of disease, including depression and mental health disorders. There are countless studies on the known benefits of exercise for cognitive function, mood, and even increasing IQ.

Acute bouts of exercise make us more resilient to stress. It signals our bodies to turn on its antioxidant producing factories and to unleash swarms of feel-good endorphins, thereby giving our bodies lots of loving signals for our cell membranes. Exercise produces free radicals, which are harmful waste products, but at the same time it increases the scavenging of free radicals. So it leaves with a net positive effect on the body. When free radicals exceed antioxidants, acute inflammation occurs. This is "the pump," muscle fatigue, and soreness associated with exercise.[2]

However, not all exercise is created equal. Exercise can quickly become a chronic stress on the body when we fail to allow muscle cells and the nervous system time to recover. Then free radicals can begin to pile up, and scavenging begins to fall behind. Measuring the volume and intensity of exercise is very important to quantify. Over-trained athletes have much higher levels of oxidative stress and diminished beneficial response to exercise-induced stress.

What follows overtraining may be caused by systemic inflammation: negative effects on the central nervous system, depressed mood, and even messing with neurohormonal signaling. Overtraining can cause an increase in the dreadful cytokines, which may act on the hypothalamic centers that act on sick-like behavior, causing mood changes. Prolonged muscle injuries prevent glucose into the muscles. This is a shortcut to increasing muscle aches, pains, and fatigue associated with autoimmunity.[3]

Usually when people train, they have a goal in mind of something they would like to improve upon. Performance increases are achieved through incrementally increasing training loads or intensity. In order to recover from a training session, you must go through a period of complete rest from exercise. Muscle tissue have microtears that need to be mended and waste products must be recycled. Many athletes follow a concept of overreaching, which is the practice of accumulating some level of mild chronic muscle damage that actually allows them to bounce back stronger and higher performing than would be without this method. It is my personal opinion that an individual with autoimmune disease who is not training for a gold medal in Taekwondo, steer away from overreaching principles and keep it simple with acute exercise loads followed by robust recovery. This eliminates the fine line between therapeutic exercise and overtraining syndrome. Keep exercise on your team in fighting against your autoimmune disease.

Unfortunately, my concept of overtraining was not mature, as I was an ex-wrestler and had the mentality to always work harder. Years later I learned not to work harder, but smarter. Early on, I had not yet discovered much of what I would learn in exercise science.

I remember when I was a freshman undergrad, and I was aspiring to break the 24-hour chin-up record. I was clocking in thousands of repetitions a week, eventually getting 1,000 chin-ups in 90 minutes during training. One day I was super excited because I'd be doing my first 3-hour pull-up workout and I awaited the personal barriers I'd break that would bring me one step closer to my goal of a world record. I was steady on pace to hit 1,800 repetitions in 3 hours; however, my right rotator cuff had different plans and gave out on me at 82 minutes. I tore it, and to be honest it wasn't the same for many years after. It doesn't take a rocket scientist to know that it might have happened due to the excessive stress I had put on my body.

My senior year of college I was chasing yet another record—this time a deadlift record. It was brute strength task, completely different than the endurance feat from 3 years prior. I had pulled 520 pounds in training at a body weight of 165 pounds, which was more than the standing record. So a few months out, I signed up for a meet. Then while lifting heavy one day in training, I felt my lower back light up in sharp pain. I dropped the weight instantaneously. I was in shock when I later learned that I had ruptured a disk in my back and that lifting absurdly dense weights was not something in my near future.

Both of those stories illustrate something. I did not injure myself randomly; it was an accumulation of training over months and months. I did not respect my body's recovery. This may have very well been a hardy amount of stress in my bank. The lesson here is that although I understand you might not be chasing world records, it is not the time to be a hero in the gym with a friend or to be a weekend warrior. This is the time to get only the right doses of exercise to yield the maximum benefits.

Another form of chronic exercise is chronic cardio. For some reason, running a marathon has earned the reputation of being one of the healthiest things for your body. In reality, it can be devastating to one's stress levels and hormone levels. Research studies have indicated that marathon runners who competed with the most frequency had higher levels of scar tissue and calcification in the heart![4] Chronic cardio and overtraining has also been shown to make the gut more permeable. It gives you temporary leaky gut![5] Even with moderate exercise, you should consider avoiding a large meal post exercise.

Multiple Sclerosis is a special case in that individuals don't want to overheat because it can trigger symptoms. Aerobic exercise training with low to moderate intensity can result in the improvement of aerobic fitness and reduction of fatigue in MS patients who are affected by mild or moderate disability. These patients are especially susceptible to exercise-related fatigue, heat intolerance, and falling.[6] MS and other neurologic autoimmune patients should instead place emphasis on balance and coordination modes of exercise to build up the nervous system.

The most common autoimmune disease, Rheumatoid Arthritis, is distinguished by joint pain and the wasting away of muscle tissue. These patients also are more likely to suffer from cardiovascular disease. The inactivity associated with RA makes the effects of the disease worse. Apart from the general effects of exercise previously mentioned in the general population, exercise has been shown to have specific health benefits in people with RA. Findings from randomized controlled trials show that properly designed physical exercise programs include improved cardiorespiratory fitness and cardiovascular health, increased muscle mass, reduced fat, improved strength, and physical functioning—all of which are achieved without flaring of the disease in joints.[7]

I understand it may be scary for people to exercise when they are in pain. But it is therapeutic as long as you are exploring pain-free ranges of motion. Exercise allows for the natural release of painkillers, and movement is tremendously important for preserving joint health. A joint that does not move loses its ability to move, and on a cellular level it speeds up the process of degeneration. Range of movement and flexibility are also improved as a result of exercise, thereby reducing movement limitations. Joint lubrication is enhanced, further acting to promote the health of an arthritic joint. More specifically, after long periods of inactivity, synovial fluid is squeezed out from between the two surfaces of a joint, resulting in contact between the areas of cartilage. When movement is resumed, the mechanism of fluid film lubrication is reactivated.[8]

Resistance training will increase not only muscle mass, but bone density loses from Rheumatoid Arthritis. Muscle, cartilage, and tendons are all made of the same stuff, but in different ratios. They all speak the same language, the language of pressure. If you input a directional pressure into a muscle or joint, it will lay down collagen into that specific directional. This can be hacked to build up the joints and muscles most pertinent to you.

Water-based exercise has also been studied in Rheumatoid Arthritis. Just 2, 30-minute sessions for 4 weeks of hydrotherapy have been shown to significantly reduce joint tenderness, improve knee range of movement, and improve emotional and psychological well-being in patients.

Dancing is another form of aerobic exercise that has reported improvements in aerobic power as well as positive changes in depression, anxiety, and fatigue, without increasing disease activity. Doctors should prescribe going to the disco!

The optimum exercise program for Rheumatoid Arthritis patients would include both aerobic and resistance training. The main cause of death in RA patients is poor cardiovascular health, so the requirement of aerobic exercise is crucial. The addition of strengthening exercises helps to mitigate rheumatoid cachexia and other musculoskeletal and joint health issues, and it induces substantial improvements in physical function and the ability to perform activities of daily living.[9]

Hydrotherapy was also studied in Multiple Sclerosis and Fibromyalgia patients. Forty sessions of aquatic exercise improved pain, spasms, disability, fatigue, depression, and autonomy in patients with MS.[10] In Fibromyalgia patients there were positive outcomes for pain, tender points, and health status.[11] Water buoyancy is going to reduce the weight that joints, bones, and muscles have to bear, and the warmth and pressure of water also reduces swelling and reduces load on painful joints, thereby promoting muscle relaxation.

There are a few different strategies that can be taken in order to exercise safely and efficiently with autoimmune disease. Isometric exercise is the act of statically contracting a muscle without movement of the joint. They are often safe for those patients who are inflamed or in a flare up. Isometrics do not have joint shear or muscle tears so there is very little inflammatory response.

There are many ways to increase the difficulty of an exercise. You can increase the load or the volume, and decrease rest or stability, etc.; another way is blood flow restriction (BFR) bands. BFR bands are a rehab/exercise modality that occlude blood in either the arms or legs. This training model requires the use of inflatable cuffs or bands that are placed at the proximal ends of the upper arms or thighs to restrict blood flow, whereby the external pressure applied is sufficient to maintain arterial inflow while occluding the venous outflow distal to the occlusion site. This results in a hypoxic environment that enhances the training effect in exercising muscle. BFR bands are a great way for individuals with joint pain to lift very light loads while also getting the benefits of exercise. Blood flow restriction (BFR) combined with low-intensity strength training has been shown to increase skeletal muscle mass and strength in a variety of populations. BFR results in a robust metabolic stress, which is hypothesized to induce muscle growth via increased recruitment of fast-twitch muscle fibers, a greater endocrine response, and/or enhancing the cellular swelling contribution to the hypertrophic process. It was observed that BFR generated a higher production of vascular endothelial growth factor (building blood vessels) and growth hormone when compared with the control.[12]

Systemic Autoimmune Myopathies (SAMs) are a heterogeneous group of rare systemic autoimmune diseases that primarily affect skeletal muscles. It was demonstrated that low-intensity strength training combined with partial blood flow restriction was a safe and effective method of increasing muscle strength, function, muscle mass, and significant improvements in the quality of life of patients.[13] In a study on women with Rheumatoid Arthritis, the group training with BFR bands had a significantly greater increase in strength and had 0 cases of injury, while in the control group 50 percent of the subjects endured exercise-induced pain.[14]

Oxygen utilization is a good indicator for chronic degenerative diseases. It is not about how much oxygen you bring in but rather how efficiently your body can use it. There is a marker called VO2 max, which is the maximum amount of oxygen your body is able to utilize during exercise. VO2 max happens to also be a predictor for longevity and all-cause mortality.[15] Fitness training can be used to increase your body's ability to use oxygen, especially under stress.

There are many different forms of exercise from which an individual with autoimmune disease can benefit. The most effective would be a combination of cardiovascular, resistance, and flexibility training. The approach may vary for each person and each disease. However, there is no question that signaling the muscles of your body to increase in strength and resilience is going to be positive in the right dosages. This is something you can work alongside a personal trainer or exercise physiologist.

NOTES

1   Centers for Disease Control and Prevention. (2021, June 11). *FASTSTATS - exercise or physical activity*. Centers for Disease Control and Prevention. Retrieved from https://www.cdc.gov/nchs/fastats/exercise.htm.

2   Yavari, A.; Javadi, M.; Mirmiran, P.; Bahadoran, Z. (2015, March). *Exercise-induced oxidative stress and dietary antioxidants*. Asian journal of sports medicine. Retrieved from https://www.ncbi.nlm.nih.gov/pmc /articles/PMC4393546.

3   Kreher, J. B. and Schwartz, J. B. (2012, March). *Overtraining syndrome: A practical guide*. Sports health. Retrieved from https://www.ncbi.nlm.nih .gov/pmc/articles/PMC3435910.

4   Reynolds, G. (2017, July 19). *The toll of exercise on the heart (and why you may not need to worry)*. The New York Times. Retrieved from https:// www.nytimes.com/2017/07/19/well/move/the-toll-of-exercise-on-the -heart-and-why-you-may-not-need-to-worry.html.

5   Zuhl, M.; Schneider, S.; Lanphere, K.; Conn, C.; Dokladny, K.; Moseley, P. (n.d.). *Exercise regulation of intestinal tight junction proteins*. British journal of sports medicine. Retrieved from https://pubmed.ncbi.nlm.nih .gov/23134759.

6   Halabchi, F.; Alizadeh, Z.; Sahraian, M. A.; Abolhasani, M. (2017, Sept. 16). *Exercise prescription for patients with multiple sclerosis; potential benefits and practical recommendations*. BMC neurology. Retrieved from https://www.ncbi.nlm.nih.gov/pmc/articles/PMC5602953.

7   Cooney, J. K.; Law, R.-J.; Matschke, V.; Lemmey, A. B.; Moore, J. P.; Ahmad, Y.; Jones, J. G.; Maddison, P.; Thom, J. M. (2011, Feb. 13). *Benefits of exercise in rheumatoid arthritis*. Journal of aging research. Retrieved from https://www.ncbi.nlm.nih.gov/pmc/articles/PMC3042669.

8   Ingram, K. R.; Wann, A. K. T.; Angel, C. K.; Coleman, P. J.; Levick, J. R. (2008, March 15). *Cyclic movement stimulates hyaluronan secretion into the synovial cavity of rabbit joints*. The Journal of physiology. Retrieved from https://www.ncbi.nlm.nih.gov/pmc/articles/PMC2375686.

9   Cooney, J. K.; Law, R.-J.; Matschke, V.; Lemmey, A. B.; Moore, J. P.; Ahmad, Y.; Jones, J. G.; Maddison, P.; Thom, J. M. (2011, Feb. 13). *Benefits of exercise in rheumatoid arthritis*. Journal of Aging Research. Retrieved from https://www.hindawi.com/journals/jar/2011/681640.

10 Castro-Sánchez, A. M.; Matarán-Peñarrocha, G. A.; Lara-Palomo, I.; Saavedra-Hernández, M.; Arroyo-Morales, M.; Moreno-Lorenzo, C. (n.d.). *Hydrotherapy for the treatment of pain in people with multiple sclerosis: A randomized controlled trial*. Evidence-based complementary and alternative medicine : eCAM. Retrieved from https://pubmed.ncbi .nlm.nih.gov/21785645.

11 Zamunér, A. R.; Andrade, C. P.; Arca, E. A.; Avila, M. A. (2019, July 3). *Impact of water therapy on pain management in patients with fibromyalgia: Current perspectives*. Journal of pain research. Retrieved from https:// www.ncbi.nlm.nih.gov/pmc/articles/PMC6613198.

12   Rossi, F. E.; de Freitas, M. C.; Zanchi, N. E.; Lira, F. S.; Cholewa, J. M. (2018, Oct. 9). *The role of inflammation and immune cells in blood flow restriction training adaptation: A Review.* Frontiers in physiology. Retrieved from https://www.ncbi.nlm.nih.gov/pmc/articles/PMC6189414/#B25.

13   de Oliveira, D. S.; Misse, R. G.; Lima, F. R.; Shinjo, S. K. (2018, May 24). *Physical exercise among patients with systemic autoimmune myopathies.* Advances in Rheumatology. Retrieved from https://advancesinrheumatology.biomedcentral.com/articles/10.1186/s42358-018-0004-1.

14   *Low-load resistance training with blood flow restriction benefits women with ra.* rheumatology.medicinematters.com. (2019, May 10). Retrieved from https://rheumatology.medicinematters.com/rheumatoid-arthritis-/physical-activity/low-load-resistance-training-with-blood-flow-restriction-benefit/16713960.

15   M;, S. B. B. (n.d.). *Survival of the fittest: VO 2 Max, a key predictor of longevity?* Frontiers in bioscience (Landmark edition). Retrieved from https://pubmed.ncbi.nlm.nih.gov/29293447.

CHAPTER 10

Healing Modalities

SHVITZING IN A SAUNA, sequestering in a hyperbaric oxygen chamber, and bathing in various light frequencies all have something in common: They are modalities that can be beneficial for managing and accelerating repair from autoimmune disease. This is where modern technology can be used as a tool for increasing the human health span. This chapter dives into various modalities that have been shown to improve symptoms associated with autoimmune disease.

Sauna

First is a therapy everyone has heard of: the sauna. The use of the sauna includes going into a heated room and inducing a mild form of hyperthermia. It has been used by many ancient cultures and its therapeutic effects are now backed by research. The increase in core temperature sets off a cascade of events including hormonal, cardiovascular, and cytoprotective mechanisms that make the body more resilient to stress.[1] The body sustains a hormetic response leading to a production of antioxidants; the physiological responses to sauna use are very similar to those experienced during exercise of moderate to vigorous intensity. Sauna is an excellent choice for those who have too much joint pain to exercise or other physical limitations due to autoimmune disease.[2]

In a study done on Rheumatoid Arthritis and Ankylosing Spondylitis patients, infrared sauna treatment had statistically significant short-term beneficial effects without any side effects. Another study effectively decreased pain in tender spots of Fibromyalgia subjects.[3, 4]

A sauna session can last 10–30 minutes depending on the temperature and resilience to the heat. Heat shock proteins are cell receptors that are responsible for cellular processes such as immune function; increased expression of heat shock proteins plays a role in repairing damaged protein structures in degenerative diseases.[5] Heat shock proteins have been shown to be particularly inhibited in certain autoimmune diseases.[6] The sauna is famed for activating heat shock proteins. Other great ways to stimulate them are through fasting and hypoxia (transient absence of oxygen).

Sauna also boosts our favorite chemical messenger, IL-10, to attack chronic inflammation.[7, 8] Your system will also be flooded with feel-good neurotransmitters and painkillers, which is an added bonus. One study found a fivefold increase in growth hormone production in subjects who alternated between sauna and cooling.[9] Some heavy metals and other environment toxins are excreted in sweat: aluminum, cadmium, cobalt, lead, BPA, PCBs, and phthalates.[10, 11, 12] Environmental toxins can be triggers and added stressors on our bodies.

It is very important to hydrate properly when using the sauna and to replenish electrolytes lost through sweating. You can try to seek out gyms that also have saunas or steam showers, which have similar effects. High heat can make symptoms associated with Multiple Sclerosis worse, so for individuals with this condition, skip the sauna. Hot baths are another great way to get heat exposure if you don't have access to a sauna, though they do not have as profound as an effect. You can try stacking the hot bath with Epsom salt to relax the muscles and joints.

UV Therapy

Epidemiology research shows that greater vitamin D levels are associated with a lower risk of certain autoimmune diseases including Multiple Sclerosis, Type 1 Diabetes, Rheumatoid Arthritis, Crohn's disease, Lupus, and Psoriasis.[13] Ultraviolet light stimulates your body's natural production of vitamin D, which plays an important role in your immune system and acts as a hormone in the body. Vitamin D also modulates the actions of regulatory T cells in beneficial ways.

So, as expected, the farther away from the equator that you live, the greater the risk of those selective autoimmune diseases.[14] If you are in a season or in a part of the world with sun exposure, it is important to try and get at least 30 minutes of sun exposure every day. Most humans in Western society don't get enough sunlight except on rare occasions such as beach days or vacations, where they have not built resilience to the sun and it becomes a harsh stress on the body. Proper dosages of UVA/UVB is needed for humans to function optimally.

If you don't live in a sunny latitude, you may want to consider heliotherapy or phototherapy. Tanning beds don't usually have the full spectrum of wavelengths found in sunlight, such as red and near-infrared light that protect against sun damage. Therefore, the therapeutic dose and length of exposure of light you receive from a tanning bed should be minimized. The importance of taking the Goldilocks approach to sun exposure is seen in Lupus patients: Too much sun will exacerbate the symptoms, too little sun will not, but a proper dose can provide symptom relief.[15] In individuals with Fibromyalgia, sunbathing creates a pain relief effect after exposure to UV light.[16] There are likely more feel-good peptides produced when humans are exposed to the sun, causing us to crave it.

Red Light / Infrared Light

The laser was invented in 1960; however, it wasn't until later in the decade that the laser was discovered to have therapeutic value. Laser stands for light amplification by stimulated emission of radiation. Red light therapy (RLT) delivers various wavelengths of light that stimulate a healing effect on the body. The different waveforms include red light, near-infrared, and far-infrared wave spectrums. Red and near-infrared waveforms energize the mitochondria at a cellular level. Red light is the wavelength between 620–700 nm. The infrared spectrum, which we cannot see with the human eye, ranges from 700nm–10,000 nm. Infrared is split up into ranges: near-, middle-, and far-infrared. The therapeutic range is from 700nm–1400nm. Near-infrared penetrates the body more deeply than red light; however there is also heat associated with this wavelength. So you wouldn't want to use infrared waves over a hot inflamed area—red light would be more appropriate in this circumstance. One solution is to use a flashing infrared light so less heat is produced. The light upregulates mitochondria to produce more ATP, which in return is effective at reducing pain and inflammation, increasing collagen production in the skin, and aiding in muscle recovery.[17] Red light and near-infrared light promote antioxidant production and reduce oxidative stress associated with pain and inflammation. They also increase circulation, which will allow injured tissues to bathe in more oxygen for healing.[18, 19, 20] RLT has had significant effectiveness in studies on Fibromyalgia patients,[21, 22] Raynaud's phenomenon,[23] Rheumatoid Arthritis,[24] Bell's palsy,[25] Multiple Sclerosis,[26] and Autoimmune Thyroditiis.[27] As you recall, the thymus is the organ that destroys hyperactive delinquent T cells. The thymus also radically atrophies as we age. Red light therapy can help prevent the atrophy of our immune system's gatekeeper.[28]

Red lights bulbs or panels can be purchased for at-home use. Not all red lights are created equal, though, so be sure to research a reputable brand and not to shine the light over any abnormal growths. Chiropractic or Physical Therapy offices can have more powerful lasers for joint-specific usage. Treatment time usually lasts 10–15 minutes.

Blood Irradiation

In the Soviet Union during the early 1980s, intravenous laser therapy began experimentation. This therapy occurs when light is shined into the blood stream via a portal into a patient's vein. There are many color wavelengths that can be used, all for different effects; different color wavelengths produce different effects. Much of the exogenous light on skin is reflected, refracted, or scattered, never making it deep into our anatomy. The blue, yellow, green, and red light all have different biological effects when they interact with our cells. This treatment has also been shown to have positive immunologic activity on the blood, improved oxygen supply, and decreased CRP.[29, 30]

Generally, the light is administered individually to the blood cells via the port into the vein. Each wavelength is administered for about 10 minutes each and is applied using very low power levels of 1–3 mW. This is done through use of a machine specifically designed to trigger the production of light. Typically, treatments are scheduled for 3–5 times per week with a total of up to 10 treatments.

Cryotherapy

Cryotherapy is the act of cooling your entire body. This can be accomplished via a cold bath, cold shower, or a cryotherapy chamber. Cryotherapy chambers use liquid nitrogen as the cooling medium and can drop down to temperatures of -300°F. The treatment only lasts about 2–3 minutes.

Cryotherapy has been shown to decrease pain in patients with Rheumatoid Arthritis, Ankylosing Spondylitis, and Fibromyalgia.[31, 32] The pain relief found in the study, however, was short-lived. So perhaps getting a daily dose of full body cold is warranted.

Local liquid nitrogen cryotherapy has been shown to help in the regrowth of hair in individuals with Alopecia[33] and Vitiligo.[34]

Cryotherapy decreases the pain while allowing the person to get more ranges of motion in physical exercise, which further increases their functionality. In addition, the acute stress of the cold ramps up the body's antioxidant production. During my experiences with cryotherapy, as I exited the frigid tank, a euphoric coat of energy surrounded my body. Prolonged cold exposure, however, is likely to depress the immune system.

It is hard to talk about the benefits of the cold without mentioning Wim Hof, an individual who holds the world record for spending the longest time in an ice bath. He is famed for popularizing a breathing technique that is now coined the Wim Hof Method. I am not going to go into detail about his breathing method in this book, but the goal of the exercises is to create a state of hypoxia, or a shortage of oxygen. This also is an acute stress on the body. Combine the Wim Hof breaths with a cold exposure, and you create a synergistic immune modulator effect. When Wim Hof breaths were tested in the lab, they were shown to increase anti-inflammatory mediators by 200 percent, and pro-inflammatory mediators were 50 percent lower.[35] Furthermore, hypoxic training stimulates the production of a hormone called erythropoietin, EPO, which increases the production of oxygen carrying red blood cells. So hypoxic training actually boosts your baseline oxygen bioavailability.[36] The breaths were also shown to activate parts of the brain associated with pain suppression.[37] Breaths are not to be done alone in bodies of water for safety reasons. Cold exposure can be contrasted with hot showers or baths, switching back and forth from cold exposure to warm exposure.

The Art of Breathing

Here is a therapy that is 100 percent free! It is something you can harness from your own body/breath work. Many individuals have lost their congenital ability to breathe efficiently. It has been derailed by chronic stress, leaky gut, and a lack of exertion. We chest breathe instead of belly breathe. We breathe more often and with larger boluses of air, but we absorb less oxygen. Worst of all, we chronically mouth breathe instead of by design through the nose.

The main determinant of how much oxygen can be utilized by your body is directly correlated with the amount of CO_2 in your blood. One notion that may be counterintuitive is that carbon dioxide is actually highly beneficial to humans. The acidity of CO_2 stimulates an immediate release of oxygen from hemoglobin to the tissues of the body. This is referred to as the Bohr effect.[38] Hemoglobin is a protein within red blood cells that is responsible for carrying oxygen,[39] which illuminates the importance of proper amounts of CO_2 in the blood for optimal oxygen unloading. With this being said, too much CO_2 also has its side effects.

The surface area of the alveoli in your lungs is about the size of a tennis court.[40] This amazing efficiency saturates blood oxygen levels up, almost maximally, to between 95–99 percent in most individuals.[41] In fact, at rest, 75 percent of oxygen is exhaled without having been used. So deeper breaths of air won't actually diffuse more oxygen into the blood, but they will force more CO_2 out of the lungs. In the absence of lung pathologies, the primary stimulus of the brain to breathe is when CO_2 levels are over a certain threshold.[42] CO_2 is considered to be a waste product from energy production; however, the body actually retains a certain amount of it during exhale. CO_2 is not only responsible for the unloading of O_2, but it also opens the airway and blood vessels. The absence of CO_2 decreases blood flow proportionally.

The main condition preventing optimal CO_2 levels is chronic overbreathing. Overbreathing can be described as breathing that is heavy, deep, asynchronous, loud, and without pause. Chronic overbreathing occurs from breathing in more volume of air than the body requires, which then results in excess CO_2 being expelled from the lungs, which drives down the amount of usable oxygen to tissues. While this may not be concerning during short bouts of intense exercise, it has profound effects over the long haul. Long-term, your body adapts by becoming more sensitive to lower levels of CO_2, thereby lowering the brain's autonomic threshold for CO_2, and continuing the status quo of deeper and more frequent breaths without more O_2 availability. The goal should be to become more CO_2 tolerant so that the body is more efficient at breathing. This overbreathing syndrome can affect individuals differently, some developing hyperventilation, others chronic fatigue and asthma, and in some it may be another stressor in the pot of autoimmunity.

The strategy we take towards breathing can influence CO_2 levels in our bodies. Breaths should sound quiet, controlled, and rhythmic versus heavy, deep, and with a pause in between breaths. Being able to deliver more oxygen throughout days, weeks, and months to our organs, joint lining, and other tissues, is going to be a big driver in the war against autoimmune disease.

Humans are designed to spend most of our resting and sleeping time breathing through our noses. Mouth breathing is reserved for fight-or-flight situations, so chronic mouth breathing will activate this system often. As referenced in Chapter 6, chronic activation of the sympathetic nervous system is going to rattle the immune system out of homeostasis. The nose is designed to cause a turbulence within the air so it can be filtered, humidified, and warmed before entering the lungs. Nose breathing brings the nitric oxide that is produced in the sinuses into your lungs, thereby dilating the blood vessels and airways, making it more efficient to breathe.[43]

Another qualm of mouth breathing is it has deleterious effects to the oral microbiome. The oral microbiome is the second most diverse in the body behind the gut, with over 700 species. Forty-five percent of the bacteria in the mouth are found in the gut. Every time you swallow, you are seeding your gut with fungi, bacteria, and viruses. The oral microbiome will have profound effects on gut microbiome and thereby play a role in leaky gut. Immune dendritic cells are found throughout the oral mucosa, and the immune system can be activated or suppressed by the milieu of bacteria in the oral cavity. Sleeping with your mouth open changes the environment in your mouth enough to cause a shifting in the bacteria populations—and enough to cause morning breath.

Colonies of S. mutans, the bacteria responsible for cavities in teeth is linked to allergies and asthma. S. mutans is increased via excessive mouth breathing, which is what leads to accumulation of dental plaque. Periodontal disease then goes on to predispose Rheumatoid Arthritis.[44] Studies have been able to link two events in history when our oral microbiome changed in a monumental way: the Neolithic and Industrial revolutions.[45] Two focal points when the human diet took a turn for the worse.

Positive Ways to Cultivate the Oral Biome

Oil pulling has been used as a part of Ayurvedic medicine for thousands of years, whereby coconut oil is swished around the mouth for 5–20 minutes in the morning on an empty stomach. This is to be thought of as a prebiotic for the oral microbiome. (Make sure to spit the oil into a cup when done.) Different oils can be used. It has been shown to kill the harmful bacteria linked to plaque[46] and bad breath.[47]

Oil pulling has been shown to be just as effective as oral mouthwash.[48] I'd like to see more research on the type of species that populate the mouth as a result of antiseptic alcohol-based mouthwash. It does decrease the bad bacteria, but I have concerns about the side effects and the possibility of nuking the whole biome. Tongue scraping is another effective measure for altering the oral biome. The act of cleaning or scraping of the tongue positively influences the tongue biome and is recommended by the American Dental Association.[49]

The technique that can be used for scraping the tongue is to use a tongue scraper and start as far back on the tongue as is comfortable and then move forward. Try and scrape the entire surface area of the tongue. Oil pulling and tongue scraping are to be used as an adjunctive with brushing and flossing, with the biggest lever being diet for creating a harmonious biome.

Furthermore, mouth breathing will activate upper chest breathing where your chest expands and hyperactivates the upper trapezius muscle, which may contribute to a tightening of the muscle. This is why stress is often associated with tight trapezius muscles. Chest breathing brings in greater volumes of air when compared to belly breathing. To the contrary, nose breathing allows for more fluid belly breathing. Belly breathing stimulates the movement of the diaphragm, which helps circulate the lymphatic systems, which is responsible for detoxification of the body. Belly breathing stimulates the parasympathetic nervous system.[50]

Once I've learned about a new scientific principle, I like to cross-check it with our ancestral wiring that has been untethered by the modern world. I do this by looking at the work of individuals who study modern-day communities or tribes that are relatively uninfluenced by modern diet and lifestyle. One great example of the switch from nasal breathing to mouth breathing is when Dr. Weston Price studied Gaelic people living on one of the Hebrides islands off the coast of Scotland. The offspring of one generation became mouth breathers after switching from their ancestral diet to modern processed foods.[51] Is it because modern foods caused leaky gut, thereby stimulating allergies/asthma to clog the nasal passage forcing mouth breathing?

Aside from humans, most forms of wildlife in the animal kingdom are strictly nasal breathers aside from eating, drinking, and cooling body temperature. Modern-day hunter-gatherers, such as the Tarahumara, don't just nasal breathe at rest but also during long extended hunts while chasing prey.[52, 53] Mouth breathing in adolescents causes malformation of the jaw and skull so that the palate is too small to fit adult teeth, thereby forcing them into different directions. And yet animals have perfect teeth unless their noses are plugged, causing the same dental destiny found in humans.

Ways to Improve CO_2 Tolerance

- Switch from mouth breathing to nasal breathing.
- Switch from chest breathing to belly breathing.
- Improve tolerance through training.
- Simulate high-altitude training.

To start, you must become conscious of the way you breathe. Set reminders, and during your meditations focus on slow, deep nasal breathings into your belly. If you are a chronic mouth breather this may irritate the nasal cavity at first, but then your body will adapt to the new movement. Various light mouth tapes can be used at nighttime to begin to train you to breathe through your nose throughout the entire night. Sympathetically driven breathing may be stimulated during sports events, high-intensity workouts, or hunting because more air volume will allow for greater force production during explosive movements. This is normal and advantageous.

For more programming and CO_2 tolerance training check out *The Oxygen Advantage* by Patrick McCowen.[54]

Hyperbaric Oxygen Therapy

Under normal conditions at sea level, oxygen makes up 21 percent of the air we breathe. We inhale 2.4 pounds of oxygen per hour. Oxygen is a rate-limiting molecule in many pathways in the body including the production of energy and healing.

Hyperbaric oxygen therapy (HBOT) entails pressurized chambers fed with 100 percent oxygen, which, by itself, won't have much therapeutic effect considering that your blood is already saturated with oxygen. However, by pressurizing the chamber, this allows for more oxygen to be dissolved into the blood, 10–20 times more, which therefore increases your body's metabolism and ability to heal. Generally, as stated, our blood is at 95–99 percent oxygen capacity. In addition, 98.5 percent of oxygen transportation to hungry cells is bound to red blood cells. There is also the 1.5 percent of oxygen that hitches a ride via the blood stream unbound to blood vessels.[55] The latter is the transportation system targeted with HBOT.

HBOT is best used as a cumulative effect over many sessions. Many studies use 40 sessions as a standard and claim that it is most effective when sessions are used consecutively, 5 times per week. Generally, a patient may be in the chamber between 1–2 hours. Most of the studies are performed on the medical-grade, hard-shell chambers. The hard shell is needed to achieve higher-pressure loads. The soft shell does not reach the higher dose of the hard-shell chambers, but it may be beneficial for healthy individuals who are looking to optimize. Soft-cell chambers can be purchased for home use.

There are some risks to HBOT, including a 1 in 10,000 chance of having a seizure, earaches, temporary changes in vision, or lung damage in those with preexisting lung complications.

HBOT upregulates natural production and mobilization of stem cells. It can push stimulated stem cells into the blood stream and will deposit them in places of the body that need healing. In the case of autoimmune disease, this can be the joints, the gut, or other organs. Successful HBOT trials have been performed for Crohn's disease,[56] Scleroderma,[57] Rheumatoid Arthritis,[58] and Fibromyalgia.[59]

Grounding / Earthing / PEMF

Earthing, also known as grounding, is the act of living in contact with Earth's surface. In today's world we are more alienated from the earth than ever before. Reconnecting to the Earth has profound health benefits. The Earth's surface has a net negative electric charge and is continuously resupplied from lightning strikes caused by the buildup of opposite charges. Our environment interacts with us through electromagnetic forces. In fact, organisms can be thought of as electromagnetic batteries. Our bodies are a vast network of electrical circuits that receive and transmit energy in the form of electrons. Our muscles, nervous system, and even immune cells are all instructed by electrical impulses.

For most of human history, people walked barefoot and slept on the ground. Our feet are meant to be in touch with the earth. The sole of the foot has more nerve endings per square inch than any other part of the body.[60] Perhaps one of the functions of this was to absorb energy from the earth's electromagnetic current. Electrons flow into humans as a form of diffusion; they move from an area of high concentration to one of lower concentration.[61] When the body becomes completely grounded to the Earth's electrical charge, electrons also could flow back. Most importantly, grounding reduces dirty electricity currents from unnatural technological electromagnetic fields on the body.

Once shoes appeared on the scene, archaeology saw atrophying of the bones in our feet.[62]

During the early days of our species, Homo sapiens left the trees to sleep on the ground, and from there elevated beds didn't reappear until several thousand years ago in ancient Egypt.[63] We have pivoted from our evolutionary crafted environment by now living in houses, buildings, wearing shoes, walking on pavement, and omitting a relationship with the Earth.

Free-flowing electrons from the feet up have a potent effect on inflammation: Electrons help neutralize free radicals, by working as an antioxidant. The evidence points towards modern humans having a deficiency of free electrons and are unable to turn off chronic inflammation from autoimmune disease. Within the outer membrane of mitochondria exits an electron transport chain, where electrons cross the membrane during the process of creating ATP, which provides energy.[64, 65] If the body is not fully saturated with electrons, you will fail to produce optimal levels of energy.

This theory has been tested in various studies. Grounding has been found to decrease pain, improve heart rate variability, and relax internal organs and inflammation.[66, 67] Earthing during sleep has been shown to normalize cortisol rhythm, thereby improving the sleep cycle.[68] Grounding also acts to prevent static electricity—the feeling you get when you touch a doorknob and get shocked.

From a modern perspective there are alternatives to walking barefoot, sleeping on the ground, or swimming in the ocean. There are bed mats, sheets, or patches that can be plugged into a grounded outlet or attached to a wire that goes into the ground outside. Furthermore, there are grounding shoes that have conductors on the bottom of the shoes that can conduct the electrons into your body.

Enemas / Suppositories

Enemas have been dated back for thousands of years, as documented by ancient Egyptians and Chinese people, and even secured a shout-out in the recovered Dead Sea Scrolls. Inserting drugs, probiotics, or other various "remedies" into the rear end has different effects than oral consumption.

A coffee enema is often used to clean out the colon in cases of chronic constipation. Claims about coffee enemas include having a detoxification effect on the body, antioxidant benefits, stimulation of bile release from the liver, and autoimmune disease management. Most of the reported benefits for coffee enemas are anecdotal. It is also worth noting that there have been reports, although rare, of colon damage after performing a coffee enema by actually causing inflammation in the rectum and colon.[69] I would like to see more research on coffee enemas going into the future. This is not something I have experimented with. I think the potential downfalls outweigh the benefits, but perhaps this depends on the individual.

Observationally, it was found that smokers have very low rates of Ulcerative Colitis. This sparked further investigation. Aside from Ulcerative Colitis, chronic cigarette smoking is a tremendous contributor for autoimmune disease. Paradoxically, the psychoactive compound in cigarettes—nicotine—has very interesting health benefits. As a compound without the toxins found in cigarettes, nicotine has been found to be protective against neural degenerative diseases and to be a potent cognitive booster. Chewing nicotine gum or taking it as a patch seemed to circumvent the harmful effects of smoking while also gaining the health benefits. Nicotine modulates T-cell activation, creating an immunosuppressive and anti-inflammatory effect. There is some evidence that due to its positive neurogenic effects, it can be useful in treating neuro autoimmune diseases such as Multiple Sclerosis or Sjogren's.[70] In some studies, transdermal nicotine has been shown to have significant positive effects in inducing remission for ulcerative colitis. Nicotine enemas have also been used in other studies with mixed results.[71]

There are also many different combinations of herbal enemas and suppositories that can be explored. Colonics is a treatment that uses large amounts of water to "flush" out the colon. This stimulates the bowels, and acts to clean the colon out. I could not find any evidence that has a mechanistic explanation for those types of combinations being beneficial for autoimmune disease. Nor could I locate any studies about using them to treat symptoms of autoimmune disease at all.

Oral probiotics have to survive harsh terrain to make it through the stomach and even then, they can deposit in places that may not be optimal, like the small intestines. On the other hand, rectal suppositories guarantee that the probiotics get to the desired location and have a greater chance at seeding into the walls. There is a lot of potential. I believe in the future we will have designer probiotics customized to your individual microbiome.

Ozone Therapy

Oxygen as a single atom is deficient in electrons. This makes the atom very unstable, and as a result, a single oxygen atom cannot exist in nature all by itself—at least not for more than a few nanoseconds. However, two oxygen atoms can join together to share electrons. This combination forms a very stable molecule referred to as O_2. This is the form of oxygen that is found in most of the air we breathe. A force such as electricity or ultraviolet light can temporarily split O_2 into two single oxygen atoms. Within nanoseconds oxygen atoms will reform back into O_2 molecules. A small percentage of them will unite in a structure of 3 oxygens (O_3), also known as ozone. The 3 oxygen atoms share the same amount of electrons that makes 2 oxygen atoms stable. The extra oxygen atom makes ozone a relatively unstable molecule. Ozone can be used as an acute stressor. It stimulates the mitochondria in your cells 10 times better than O_2 can to use the oxygen they get more efficiently.

Medical ozone is made by passing pure oxygen (O_2) through a generator designed for that purpose. As the O_2 flows through the tube, an electrical current is directed across the tube. This current breaks the O_2 molecules into separate single oxygen atoms. But as explained, these single oxygen atoms cannot exist in nature, so they immediately combine back into O_2 molecules. But a portion of them, roughly 2–3 percent, combine into a triplet of 3 oxygen atoms. This new molecule, O_3, is ozone. The longer the ozone is unused, the more of it that will revert back to O_2. If we wait too long the ozone will be gone, and all we will have is O_2.

Ozone can safely be applied to every part of the human body except the lungs. Ozone therapy increases the delivery of oxygen to the cells, oxygen utilization, and antioxidant enzymes. The oxygen that goes into an ozone generator must be pure, or contaminated oxidized molecules may be formed that could be harmful to you. There are two forms of oxygen that you can buy. One is called welding or industrial grade. The other is medical grade. Industrial grade is easier to get your hands on. There are a few different ways to absorb ozone, including: ozonating water, ear insufflation, rectal insufflation, bagging a limb, or cupping. For rectal insufflation a bag is filled, and a catheter is attached to the bag, which is then inserted rectally. The dosage and volume of ozone varies and needs to be worked up to.

The most potent treatment is the IV 10 pass blood session, when blood is pulled from your veins, ozonated, and then pumped back into the blood stream. Ozone therapy has been combined with sauna, hence the ozone sauna. The head of an individual pokes out through a hole in top of the sauna as the body lies submerged in the ozone-infused shell.

Ozone treatments have been beneficial for decreasing inflammation and stimulating membrane growth in Rheumatoid Arthritis patients,[72] increasing antioxidant defenses and anti-inflammatory cytokines in Multiple Sclerosis patients,[73] and providing beneficial effects on immune response in patients with Scleroderma.[74] One study measured gut dysbiosis changes to rectal insufflation and ozonated water at 45 and 90 days. At the end of the study, every single patient had a significant decrease in symptoms related to dysbiosis and a creation of a more homeostatic microbiome. This indicates that ozone either selectively destroys pathogenic bacteria strains or stimulates the beneficial strains.[75] Outside of these studies, most of the evidence is anecdotal. I would like to see more and better-controlled studies done in the future with ozone therapy.

Stem Cells / Exosomes

Stem cells are immature cells that have the potential to develop into any other cell in the body based on the environmental signals placed on it. They can be harvested from bone marrow, fat, or the umbilical cord. It is a constant debate within the stem cell field as to which types of stem cells are the most effective. Stem cells can be injected into the site of injury or into the blood for a systematic effect. This means that for IBD, targeting the gut would be most effective, and for Lupus, it would need more of a systematic approach. The idea is the stem cells will replace the old dysfunction cells with young healthy ones. This may only work short term if you don't follow the entire protocol of giving the stem cells positive environmental signals to grew into healthy, robust cells.

Exosomes are chemical messengers that can be stacked with stem cells and turn on and increase the effectiveness of stem cells. There is a lot of research being done in this area. Stem cells can be very expensive, but you can look to being a participant in a research study for free treatment. You can also look for trials on clinicaltrials.gov.

Thymus Activation

The thymus is the primary organ for the creation of T cells and acts as the filter for eliminating dysfunctional hyperactive T cells. Early on, the thymus begins to atrophy. In fact, it begins to decline as early as the second year of life. This diminishes the ability of the immune system surveillance. When I first learned about how young the thymus peaks, I immediately thought of how critical the first year of life is for educating the immune system for the rest of someone's life. It should be in our best interest to preserve a healthy, functioning, and active thymus gland to maintain a resilient immune system. The thymus does have the ability to regenerate,[76] so we must give it the proper signals. Thymic atrophy is correlated to micronutrient and protein deficiencies, increased levels of cortisol, and low levels of the satiation hormone leptin.

Growth hormone is one the signals that will stimulate thymocyte production. Again, this is living a healthy lifestyle of resistance training, and intermittent fasting will boost GH levels.[77]

Another way to stimulate the thymus gland is by thymus tapping. The thymus gland sits behind the sternum. There isn't any scientific evidence for or against thymus tapping, although tapping has been shown to be effective when applied to acupoints for decreasing stress and fear signals on the body.[78] Tapping had been used in eastern medicine for thousands of years. Here's how:

- Using your fingertips or the side of your fist, tap up and down about 2–3 inches along your sternum, between and above your breasts. The thymus is located behind the third rib, but any vibrations along the length of the upper sternum will stimulate it.

- Do this for 15–20 seconds and continue to take regular slow breaths.

- Repeat 1–3 times a day or during your meditation.

All the modalities discussed in this chapter can be used to help accelerate healing. However, without removing most of the triggers of autoimmune disease, they are unlikely to end the disease process. These can be used in conjunction with diet and lifestyle, and prescribed in specific individual dosages.

NOTES

1 Laukkanen, Jari A.; Laukkanen, Tanjaniina; Kunutsor, Setor K. Cardiovascular and Other Health Benefits of Sauna Bathing: A Review of the Evidence Mayo Clinic Proceedings 93, no. 8 (Aug. 2018): 1111–21. doi:10.1016/j.mayocp.2018.04.008.

2 McCarty, Mark F.; Jorge Barroso-Aranda; Francisco Contreras. *Regular thermal therapy may promote insulin sensitivity while boosting expression of endothelial nitric oxide synthase Effects comparable to those of exercise training.* Medical Hypotheses 73, no. 1 (July 2009): 103–5. doi:10.1016/j. mehy.2008.12.020.

3 Hussain, J. and Cohen, M. (2018, April 24). *Clinical effects of regular dry sauna bathing: A systematic review.* Evidence-based complementary and alternative medicine : eCAM. Retrieved from https://www.ncbi.nlm.nih .gov/pmc/articles/PMC5941775.

4 Oosterveld, F. G. J.; Rasker, J. J.; Floors, M.; Landkroon, R.; van Rennes, B.; Zwijnenberg, J.; van de Laar, M. A. F. J.; Koel, G. J. (2008, Aug. 7). *Infrared sauna in patients with rheumatoid arthritis and ankylosing spondylitis.* Clinical Rheumatology. Retrieved from https://link.springer .com/article/10.1007/s10067-008-0977-y.

5 Leak, Rehana K. Heat shock proteins in neurodegenerative disorders and aging. *Journal of Cell Communication and Signaling* 8, no. 4 (Sept. 2014): 293–310. doi:10.1007/s12079-014-0243-9.

6 Tukaj, S. and Kaminski, M. (2019, May). *Heat shock proteins in the therapy of autoimmune diseases: Too simple to be true?* Cell stress & chaperones. Retrieved from https://www.ncbi.nlm.nih.gov/pmc/articles/PMC6527538.

7 Singh, R.; K?lvraa, S.; P. Bross; Christensen, K.; Bathum, L.; Gregersen, N.; Tan, Q.; Rattan, S. I. Anti-inflammatory heat shock protein 70 genes are positively associated with human survival. *Curr. Pharm. Des.* 16, no. 7 (2010): 796–801.

8 Żychowska, Małgorzata; Nowak-Zaleska, Alicja; Chruściński, Grzegorz; Zaleski, Ryszard; Mieszkowski, Jan; Niespodziński, Bartłomiej; Tymański, Roman; Kochanowicz, Andrzej. Association of High Cardiovascular Fitness and the Rate of Adaptation to Heat Stress. *BioMed Research International* 2018 (2018): 1–6. doi:10.1155/2018/1685368.

9 Kukkonen-Harjula, K.; Oja, P.; Laustiola, K.; Vuori, I.; Jolkkonen, J.; Siitonen, S.; Vapaatalo, H. (n.d.). *Haemodynamic and hormonal responses to heat exposure in a finnish sauna bath.* European Journal of Applied Physiology. Retrieved from https://link.springer.com /article/10.1007%2FBF02330710.

10 Genius, Stephen J.; Birkholz, Detlef; Rodushkin, Ilia; Beesoon, Sanjay. Blood, Urine, and Sweat (BUS) Study: Monitoring and Elimination of Bioaccumulated Toxic Elements. *Archives of Environmental Contamination and Toxicology* 61, no. 2 (November 2010): 344–57. doi:10.1007/s00244 -010-9611-5.

11   Genuis, Stephen J.; Beesoon, Sanjay; Birkholz, Detlef; Lobo, Rebecca A.. Human Excretion of Bisphenol A: Blood, Urine, and Sweat (BUS) Study. *Journal of Environmental and Public Health* 2012 (2012): 1–10. doi:10.1155/2012/185731.

12   Genuis, Stephen J.; Beesoon, Sanjay; Birkholz, Detlef. Biomonitoring and Elimination of Perfluorinated Compounds and Polychlorinated Biphenyls through Perspiration: Blood, Urine, and Sweat Study. *ISRN Toxicology* 2013 (2013): 1–7. doi:10.1155/2013/483832.

13   Parnell, G. P.; Schibeci, S. D.; Fewings, N. L. (2018, Oct. 4). *Latitude-dependent autoimmune disease risk genes ZMIZ1 and IRF8 regulate mononuclear phagocytic cell differentiation in response to vitamin D.* OUP Academic. Retrieved from https://academic.oup.com/hmg /article/28/2/269/5115479.

14   Booth, D. R.; Ding, N.; Parnell, G. P.; Shahijanian, F.; Coulter, S.; Schibeci, S. D.; Atkins, A. R.; Stewart, G. J.; Evans, R. M.; Downes, M.; Liddle, C. (2016, June). *Cistromic and genetic evidence that the vitamin D receptor mediates susceptibility to latitude-dependent autoimmune diseases.* Genes and immunity. Retrieved from https://www.ncbi.nlm.nih.gov/pmc/articles /PMC4895389.

15   Pavel, S. (2006, March 7). *Light therapy (with UVA-1) for SLE patients: Is it a good or bad idea?* OUP Academic. Retrieved from https://academic .oup.com/rheumatology/article/45/6/653/1785119.

16   Juzeniene, A. and Moan, J. (2012, April 1). *Beneficial effects of UV radiation other than via vitamin D production.* Dermato-endocrinology. Retrieved from https://www.ncbi.nlm.nih.gov/pmc/articles/PMC3427189.

17   Hamblin M. "Mechanisms and Mitochondrial Redox Signaling in Photobiomodulation" *Photochemistry and Photobiology.* 2018, 94:199–212. 2017 Oct. 31. doi: 10.1111/php.12864)

18   Ferraresi, C.; Hamblin, M.; Parizotto N. "Low-level laser (light) therapy (LLLT) on muscle tissue: performance, fatigue and repair benefited by the power of light." Photonics Lasers Med. 2012 Nov. 1; 1(4): 267–286. doi:10.1515/plm-2012-0032.

19   Al Rashoud A. S.; Abboud, R. J.; Wang, W.; Wigderowitz, C. "Efficacy of low-level laser therapy applied at acupuncture points in knee osteoarthritis: a randomised double-blind comparative trial." Physiotherapy. 2014 Sept.; 100(3):242–8.

20   de Abreu, Emília; Chaves, M.; Rodrigues de Araújo, A.; Piancastelli, A. C. C.; Pinotti, M. "Effects of low-power light therapy on wound healing: LASER x LED." An Bras Dermatol. 2014 July–Aug.; 89(4): 616–623.

21   de Souza. R. C.; de Sousa, E. T.; Scudine, K. G.; Meira, U. M.; de Oliveira, E.; Silva, E. M.; Gomes, A. C.; Limeira-Junior, F. A. (n.d.). *Low-level laser therapy and anesthetic infiltration for orofacial pain in patients with fibromyalgia: A randomized clinical trial.* Medicina oral, patologia oral y cirugia bucal. Retrieved from https://pubmed.ncbi.nlm.nih.gov/29274162.

22   Yeh, S. W.; Hong, C. H.; Shih, M. C.; Tam, K. W.; Huang, Y. H.; Kuan, Y. C. (n.d.). *Low-level laser therapy for fibromyalgia: A systematic review*

and meta-analysis. Pain physician. Retrieved from https://pubmed.ncbi. nlm.nih.gov/31151332.

23 M;, H. M. K. R. F. C. K. (n.d.). *Low level laser therapy in primary Raynaud's phenomenon--results of a placebo controlled, double blind intervention study.* The Journal of rheumatology. Retrieved from https://pubmed.ncbi .nlm.nih.gov/15570642.

24 Brosseau, L.; Robinson, V.; Wells, G.; Debie, R.; Gam, A.; Harman, K.; Morin, M.; Shea, B.; Tugwell, P. (n.d.). *Low level laser therapy (classes I, II and III) for treating rheumatoid arthritis.* The Cochrane database of systematic reviews. Retrieved from https://pubmed.ncbi.nlm.nih .gov/16235295.

25 Rubis, L. M. (2013, Dec.). *Chiropractic management of Bell Palsy with low level laser and manipulation: A case report.* Journal of chiropractic medicine. Retrieved from https://www.ncbi.nlm.nih.gov/pmc/articles /PMC3838725.

26 Gonçalves, E. D.; Souza, P.S.; Lieberknecht, V.; Fidelis, G. S.; Barbosa, R. I.; Silveira, P. C.; de Pinho, R. A.; Dutra, R. C. (n.d.). *Low-level laser therapy ameliorates disease progression in a mouse model of multiple sclerosis.* Autoimmunity. Retrieved from https://pubmed.ncbi.nlm.nih .gov/26703077.

27 Höfling, D. B.; Chavantes, M. C.; Juliano, A. G.; Cerri, G. G.; Romão, R.; Yoshimura, E. M.; Chammas, M. C. (n.d.). *Low-level laser therapy in chronic autoimmune thyroiditis: A pilot study.* Lasers in surgery and medicine. Retrieved from https://pubmed.ncbi.nlm.nih.gov/20662037.

28 Odinokov, D. and Hamblin, M. R. (2018, Aug.). *Aging of lymphoid organs: Can photobiomodulation reverse age-associated thymic involution via stimulation of extrapineal melatonin synthesis and bone marrow stem cells?*Journal of biophotonics. Retrieved from https://www.ncbi.nlm.nih .gov/pmc/articles/PMC599560.

29 Momenzadeh, S. Abbasi, M.; Ebadifar, A.; Aryani, M.; Bayrami, J.; & Nematollahi, F. (2015). *The intravenous laser blood irradiation in chronic pain and fibromyalgia.* Journal of lasers in medical sciences. Retrieved from https://www.ncbi.nlm.nih.gov/pmc/articles/PMC4329142.

30 *Intravenous laser irradiation of blood—vielight inc.* (n.d.). Retrieved from https://vielight.com/wp-content/uploads/2017/12/Intravenous-Laser -Irradiation-of-Blood.pdf.

31 WH;, M. D. Z. C. P. W. J. (n.d.). *[whole-body cryotherapy in rehabilitation of patients with rheumatoid diseases--pilot study].* Die Rehabilitation. Retrieved from https://pubmed.ncbi.nlm.nih.gov/10832164.

32 Mooventhan, A. and Nivethitha, L. (2014, May). *Scientific evidence-based effects of hydrotherapy on various systems of the body.* North American journal of medical sciences. Retrieved from https://www.ncbi.nlm.nih.gov /pmc/articles/PMC4049052.

33 Zawar, V. P. and Karad, G. M. (2016). *Liquid nitrogen cryotherapy in recalcitrant alopecia areata: A study of 11 patients.* International journal

of trichology. Retrieved from https://www.ncbi.nlm.nih.gov/pmc/articles/PMC4830166.

34   Nuzzo, S. D. and Masotti, A. (2010, Jan. 24). *Depigmentation therapy in Vitiligo Universalis with cryotherapy and 4-hydroxyanisole.* Wiley Online Library. Retrieved from https://onlinelibrary.wiley.com/doi/epdf/10.1111/j.1365-2230.2009.03412.x.

35   Kox, M.; van Eijk, L. T.; Zwaag, J.; van den Wildenberg, J.; Sweep, F. C. G. J.; van der Hoeven, J. G.; Pickkers, P. (2014, May 20). *Voluntary activation of the sympathetic nervous system and attenuation of the innate immune response in humans.* Proceedings of the National Academy of Sciences of the United States of America. Retrieved from https://www.ncbi.nlm.nih.gov/pmc/articles/PMC4034215.

36   C;, S. H. S. H. J. E. K. U. B. (n.d.). *Role of erythropoietin in adaptation to hypoxia.* Experientia. Retrieved from https://pubmed.ncbi.nlm.nih.gov/2253723.

37   University, W. S. (n.d.). *Novel study is first to demonstrate brain mechanisms that give "the Iceman" unusual resistance to cold.* Today@Wayne. Retrieved from https://today.wayne.edu/news/2018/02/28/novel-study-is-first-to-demonstrate-brain-mechanisms-that-give-the-iceman-unusual-resistance-to-cold-6232.

38   Riggs, A. F. (n.d.). *The Bohr effect.* Annual Reviews. Retrieved from https://www.annualreviews.org/doi/pdf/10.1146/annurev.ph.50.030188.001145.

39   Hafen, B. B. (2021, Aug. 12). *Oxygen saturation.* StatPearls [Internet]. Retrieved from https://www.ncbi.nlm.nih.gov/books/NBK525974.

40   Williams, M. (1992, Jan. 18). *Forum: The Air Sacs and the tennis court—Mark Williams finds fault with some established truths.* New Scientist. Retrieved from https://www.newscientist.com/article/mg13318045-700-forum-the-air-sacs-and-the-tennis-court-mark-williams-finds-fault-with-some-established-truths.

41   Collins, J.-A.; Rudenski, A.; Gibson, J.; Howard, L.; O'Driscoll R. (2015, Sept.). *Relating oxygen partial pressure, saturation and content: The haemoglobin-oxygen dissociation curve.* Breathe (Sheffield, England). Retrieved from https://www.ncbi.nlm.nih.gov/pmc/articles/PMC4666443.

42   Brinkman, J. E. (2021, Aug. 24). *Physiology, Respiratory Drive.* StatPearls [Internet]. Retrieved from https://www.ncbi.nlm.nih.gov/books/NBK482414.

43   Lundberg, J. O.; Settergren, G.; Gelinder, S.; Lundberg, J. M.; Alving, K.; Weitzberg, E. (n.d.). *Inhalation of nasally derived nitric oxide modulates pulmonary function in humans.* Acta physiologica Scandinavica. Retrieved from https://pubmed.ncbi.nlm.nih.gov/8971255.

44   Nelson-Dooley, C. and Olmstead, S. (2005, March). *The Microbiome and Overall Health.* Prothera. Retrieved from https://www.drkarafitzgerald.com/wp-content/uploads/2015/06/2015-Oral-Microbiome-Nelson-Dooley-Olmstead.pdf.

45   Adler, C. J.; Dobney, K.; Weyrich, L. S.; Kaidonis, J.; Walker, A. W.; Haak, W.; Bradshaw, C. J. A.; Townsend, G.; Sołtysiak, A.; Alt, K. W.; Parkhill,

J.; Cooper, A. (2013, April). *Sequencing ancient calcified dental plaque shows changes in oral microbiota with dietary shifts of the neolithic and industrial revolutions.* Nature genetics. Retrieved from https://www.ncbi .nlm.nih.gov/pmc/articles/PMC3996550.

46 R;, A. S. E. P. C. (n.d.). *Effect of oil pulling on plaque induced gingivitis: A randomized, controlled, triple-blind study.* Indian journal of dental research: official publication of Indian Society for Dental Research. Retrieved from https://pubmed.ncbi.nlm.nih.gov/19336860.

47 Shanbhag, V. K. L. (2016, June 6). *Oil pulling for maintaining oral hygiene – A Review.* Journal of traditional and complementary medicine. Retrieved from https://www.ncbi.nlm.nih.gov/pmc/articles/PMC5198813.

48 Kaushik, M.; Reddy, P.; Sharma, R.; Udameshi, P.; Mehra, N.; Marwaha, A. (n.d.). *The effect of coconut oil pulling on streptococcus mutans count in saliva in comparison with chlorhexidine mouthwash.* The journal of contemporary dental practice. Retrieved from https://pubmed.ncbi.nlm .nih.gov/27084861.

49 Tribble, G. D.; Angelov, N.; Weltman, R.; Wang, B.-Y.; Eswaran, S. V.; Gay, I. C.; Parthasarathy, K.; Dao, D.-H. V.; Richardson, K. N.; Ismail, N. M.; Sharina, I. G.; Hyde, E. R.; Ajami, N. J.; Petrosino, J. F.; Bryan, N. S. (2019, March 1). *Frequency of tongue cleaning impacts the human tongue microbiome composition and enterosalivary circulation of nitrate.* Frontiers in cellular and infection microbiology. Retrieved from https:// www.ncbi.nlm.nih.gov/pmc/articles/PMC6406172.

50 Wang, S. Z.; Li, S.; Xu, X. Y.; Lin, G. P.; Shao, L.; Zhao, Y.; Wang, T. H. (n.d.). *Effect of slow abdominal breathing combined with biofeedback on blood pressure and heart rate variability in prehypertension.* Journal of alternative and complementary medicine (New York, N.Y.). Retrieved from https://pubmed.ncbi.nlm.nih.gov/20954960.

51 Price, W. A. (2020). *Nutrition and physical degeneration.* Price-Pottenger Nutrition Foundation.

52 *Airflow and performance: How athletes naturally boost performance - alabama nasal and Sinus Center, Birmingham, AL, ent.* Alabama Nasal & Sinus Center—Birmingham, Ala. (2018, February 5). Retrieved from https://alabamasinus.com/airflow-and-performance-how-athletes -naturally-boost-performance.

53 *The energetic paradox of human . . . —University of Utah.* (n.d.). Retrieved from https://carrier.biology.utah.edu/Dave's%20PDF/energetic%20 paradox.pdf.

54 McKeown, P. (2016). *The oxygen advantage: Simple, scientifically proven breathing techniques to help you become healthier, slimmer, faster, and fitter.* William Morrow, an imprint of HarperCollins Publishers.

55 Maxfield, W. S. (2017). *The oxygen cure: A complete guide to hyperbaric oxygen therapy.* Humanix Books.

56 Division of Gastroenterology and Department of Medicine. (n.d.). *Hyperbaric oxygen therapy for perineal crohn's disease : Official Journal of the American College of Gastroenterology: ACG.* LWW. Retrieved from

https://journals.lww.com/ajg/Abstract/1999/02000/Hyperbaric_Oxygen_Therapy_for_Perineal_Crohn_s.10.aspx.

57 Markus, Y. M.; Bell, M. J.; Evans, A. W. (2006, Aug. 1). *Ischemic scleroderma wounds successfully treated with hyperbaric oxygen therapy.* The Journal of Rheumatology. Retrieved from http://www.jrheum.org /content/33/8/1694.short.

58 Slade, J. B.; Potts, M. V.; Flower, A. M.; Sky, K. M.; Sit, M. T.; Schmidt, T. W. (n.d.). *Pain improvement in rheumatoid arthritis with hyperbaric oxygen: Report of three cases.* Undersea & hyperbaric medicine : Journal of the Undersea and Hyperbaric Medical Society, Inc. Retrieved from https://pubmed.ncbi.nlm.nih.gov/28763177.

59 Atzeni, F.; Casale, R.; Alciati, A.; Masala, I. F.; Batticciotto, A.; Talotta, R.; Gerardi, M. C.; Salaffi, F.; Sarzi-Puttini, P. (n.d.). *Hyperbaric oxygen treatment of fibromyalgia: A prospective observational clinical study.* Clinical and experimental rheumatology. Retrieved from https://pubmed .ncbi.nlm.nih.gov/30747099.

60 *Feet facts.* Your Foot & Ankle Specialist in Sault Ste. Marie. (n.d.). Retrieved from https://www.simardfootclinic.com/feet-facts.

61 Applewhite, R. (2005) The effectiveness of a conductive patch and a conductive bed pad in reducing induced human body voltage via the application of earth ground. European biology and Bioelectromagnetics, 1, 23-40. - references - scientific research publishing. (n.d.). Retrieved from https://www.scirp.org/(S(vtj3fa45qm1ean45vvffcz55))/reference /ReferencesPapers.aspx?ReferenceID=1449735.

62 Koerth, M. (2008, June 5). *First shoes worn 40,000 years ago.* LiveScience. Retrieved from https://www.livescience.com/4964-shoes-worn-40-000-years.html.

63 Wadley, L.; Sievers, C.; Bamford, M.; Goldberg, P.; Berna, F.; Miller, C. (n.d.). *Middle stone age bedding construction and settlement patterns at Sibudu, South Africa.* Science (New York, N.Y.). Retrieved from https:// pubmed.ncbi.nlm.nih.gov/22158814.

64 64 K;, S. P. S. (n.d.). *The neuromodulative role of earthing.* Medical hypotheses.Retrieved from https://pubmed.ncbi.nlm.nih.gov/21856083.

65 Oschman, J. L.; Chevalier, G.; Brown, R. (2015, March 24). *The effects of grounding (earthing) on inflammation, the immune response, wound healing, and prevention and treatment of chronic inflammatory and autoimmune diseases.* Journal of inflammation research. Retrieved from https://www.ncbi.nlm.nih.gov/pmc/articles/PMC4378297/#b1-jir-8-083.

66 Chevalier, G.; Sinatra, S. T.; Oschman, J. L.; Sokal, K.; Sokal, P. (2012). *Earthing: Health implications of reconnecting the human body to the Earth's surface electrons.* Journal of environmental and public health. Retrieved from https://www.ncbi.nlm.nih.gov/pmc/articles/PMC3265077.

67 Chevalier, G. and Sinatra, S.T. (2011) *Emotional stress, heart rate variability, grounding and improved autonomic tone clinical applications.* Integrative Medicine a clinician's journal, 10, 16-21. - references - scientific research publishing. (n.d.). Retrieved from https://www

.scirp.org/(S(i43dyn45teexjx455qlt3d2q))/reference/ReferencesPapers
.aspx?ReferenceID=1333064.

68   *The biologic effects of grounding the human body during . . .* (n.d.). Retrieved
     from https://www.liebertpub.com/doi/10.1089/acm.2004.10.767.

69   Lee, A. H.; Kabashneh, S.; Tsouvalas, C. P.; Rahim, U.; Khan, M. Y.;
     Anees, M.; Levine, D. (2020, Jan. 2). *Proctocolitis from Coffee Enema.*
     ACG case reports journal. Retrieved from https://www.ncbi.nlm.nih.gov
     /pmc/articles/PMC7145153/#R17.

70   Piao, W.-H.; Campagnolo, D.; Dayao, C.; Lukas, R. J.; Wu, J.; Shi, F.-
     D. (2009, June). *Nicotine and inflammatory neurological disorders.* Acta
     pharmacologica Sinica. Retrieved from https://www.ncbi.nlm.nih.gov
     /pmc/articles/PMC4002379.

71   Sandborn, W. and Tremaine, W. (1997, March). Transdermal Nicotine
     for Mildly to Moderately Active Ulcerative Colitis. Retrieved from
     https://www.acpjournals.org/doi/full/10.7326/0003-4819-126-5-
     199703010-00004?casa_token=B9pZcDV-T5wAAAAA%3Ad13bNjdh9
     3tdVItr7PPbvKIjnUNZKpwIStwz5FLMfG2_XDrLB59xrE1X8J2a1noK-
     nFbMhvM5frjjg.

72   Bozbas, G. T. (n.d.). *New Therapeutic Aproach in RHEUMATOID
     ARTHRITIS: Ozone.* ClinMed International Library. Retrieved from
     https://clinmedjournals.org/articles/ijp/international-journal-of-physiatry
     -ijp-2-007.php?jid=ijp.

73   Delgado-Roche, L.; Riera-Romo, M.; Mesta, F.; Hernández-Matos, Y.;
     Barrios, J. M.; Martínez-Sánchez, G.; Al-Dalaien, S. M. (n.d.). *Medical
     ozone promotes Nrf2 phosphorylation reducing oxidative stress and
     pro-inflammatory cytokines in multiple sclerosis patients.* European
     journal of pharmacology. Retrieved from https://pubmed.ncbi.nlm.nih
     .gov/28623000.

74   D;, N. (n.d.). *Positive effect of ozonotherapy on serum concentration of
     soluble interleukin-2 receptor and neopterin in patients with systemic
     sclerosis.* Postepy dermatologii i alergologii. Retrieved from https://
     pubmed.ncbi.nlm.nih.gov/31320847.

75   *The use of ozonated water and rectal insufflation in patients with
     INTESTINAL DYSBIOSIS: Ozone therapy.* The use of ozonated water
     and rectal insufflation in patients with intestinal dysbiosis | Ozone
     Therapy. (n.d.). Retrieved from https://www.pagepressjournals.org/index
     .php/ozone/article/view/7304/7100.

76   https://orcid.org/0000-0002-8480-7391, T. W., https://orcid.org/0000-
     0001-8383-0453, E. V., & https://orcid.org/0000-0002-9267-4584, J. T.
     (2018, Jan. 26). *Production of BMP4 by endothelial cells is crucial for
     endogenous thymic regeneration.* Science Immunology. Retrieved from
     https://www.science.org/doi/10.1126/sciimmunol.aal2736.

77   Holländer, G. A.; Krenger, W.; Blazar, B. R. (2010, Aug.). *Emerging
     strategies to boost thymic function.* Current opinion in pharmacology.
     Retrieved from https://www.ncbi.nlm.nih.gov/pmc/articles/PMC3123661.

78   Feinstein, D. (2010). Rapid treatment of PTSD: Why psychological
     exposure with acupoint tapping may be effective. *Psychotherapy: Theory,
     Research, Practice, Training, 47*(3), 385–402.

CHAPTER 11

Professional Therapies

CRACKING JOINTS, SHARP NEEDLES, and hypnotizing, oh my! This chapter explores several professional therapies that can aid in the recovery of autoimmunity. Among them are chiropractic, acupuncture, and hypnotherapy.

Chiropractic

Chiropractic is the science, art, and philosophy of delivering forces into specific restricted joints anywhere in the body, but most well known in the spine. The practice has been around for thousands of years in numerous cultures. Chiropractic has developed more into science in the last few decades, now that there is more and more research coming out on the efficacy of various treatments. Chiropractic is an art in the sense that each chiropractor you go to might have different assessments, different techniques, and different treatment protocols for a specific problem. This doesn't mean necessarily that one is superior to the other, but rather that one protocol or technique may work more efficiently with varying patient presentations.

Originally based on philosophy, chiropractic was founded as a philosophy because when it was modernized within the United States in the late 1800s, neuroscience was not yet a well-studied field. Many practitioners could not explain the mechanism as to why their patients would be relieved of pain when they were given chiropractic adjustments. The more research and discoveries within the field of neuroscience that became known, the greater the blend chiropractic came to be seen as more of a science and less of a philosophy. Although most of the research on chiropractic is in the treatment of musculoskeletal system, the philosophy and theory point to some effects that chiropractic treatment can have on the immune system. Eventually, I believe discoveries in the neuroscience space will be able to prove more concepts in chiropractic that are not available today. It is my belief that raw chiropractic care alone is not enough for long-term success, but rather mixed in with active care or physical therapies to strengthen and increase the function and resilience of the spine as well.

Earlier in the book I explained the importance of maintaining homeostasis. One aspect of homeostasis is the balance between the parasympathetic and the sympathetic nervous system as controlled by the autonomic nervous system. In a particular tissue the activation of one part of the autonomic nervous system inhibits the other.[1] In your body's pursuit of homeostasis, sensory perception provides the initial step towards homeostasis and higher neural function.[2] Sensory information is collected by special cells called mechanoreceptors in the periphery, and passes the information along to the central nervous system and autonomic nervous system. Based on the incoming signal, your body sends out a signal for it to react. Maybe it's a burning finger on the stove so you rapidly pull away even before you sense the burn, or maybe it's just giving info on how you should balance while standing. Anything that interferes with this system's ability to send information is going to knock the body out of homeostasis. And when the body is chronically out of homeostasis, it prepares a breeding ground for disease.

Traditionally in chiropractic, it was taught that practitioners were treating bones that were out of place and putting them back into place. However, in the majority of cases it's quite the opposite: It's a joint that is restricted and has lost the ability to move through its full range. There is a joint in between every vertebra in the spinal. A healthy spine is able to segment at each joint. When someone loses the ability to segment at one point in the spine, it causes hinge points and adds force at other levels of the spine. Here's the catch: both the hypomobile[3] and hypermobile[4] joints experience accelerated degeneration. The hypomobile joints are not able to get nutrients to the avascular tissues without movement, and the hypermobile joints are being abused. After someone gets a spinal fusion, the joints above and below that segment rapidly degenerate.[5] So, the goal is to restore proper movement at levels of the spine.

The purpose of a chiropractic adjustment or manipulation is to restore mobility to a restricted or hypomobile joint. A chiropractic adjustment is a form of a controlled force into a specific segment of the spine. To wrap all the concepts together, when a joint becomes restricted it alters the movement at adjacent joints and also at other joints of the body throughout the kinetic chain. A restriction can be caused by injury or microinjuries, which lead to the muscles around the injury to be guarded. Altered movement patterns place extra strain and force in certain areas causing degeneration. Degeneration causes inflammation and the release of chemical signals responsible for pain sensation. The heightened pain signal increases the sympathetic (fight-or-flight) nervous system, pushing the body out of homeostasis. Restricted joints and pain have the power to wobble the autonomic nervous system, which leads it to dial up the sympathetic nervous system, which in turn can cause increased blood pressure, heart issues, and metabolic syndrome.[6]

Vertebral Subluxation Complex

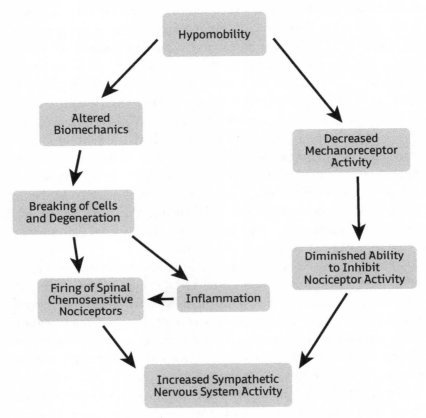

In addition to the science of chiropractic is its theoretical philosophy. Visceral or organ hypersensitivity can be caused by autonomic system dysfunction.[7] This means that altered communication is going to organs from the central nervous system. A hypersensitive organ is the hallmark of the beginning of autoimmune activity. Nerves that innervate specific muscles and organs exit at each spinal segment. Orthopedic and neurologic exams can test at what level of the spine there are compromised nerves. If a specific muscle is numb, weak, or tingly, it offers an idea of where the problem stems. However, although there are exams to test organ function and paralysis, there are no great clinical tests to measure organ performance related to spinal segment restriction versus something systematic.

Your breathing is controlled by nerves that originate from the C3, C4, and C5 spinal segments sending information to the diaphragm to breathe. This is why breaking your upper neck is lethal because you lose the ability to breathe. But this doesn't have to be an all-or-none principle. The faucet of nerve flow can be turned on all the way or to partially clogged or to just dripping. To demonstrate this analogy, a study done how on patients with high blood pressure responded to chiropractic manipulation showed that they had an immediate decrease in blood pressure that was equivalent to taking two different medications at the same time.[8] Pain stimulus in the spine produces measurable changes in sympathetic activity and nerve function, vasoconstricting and decreasing blood flow to organs.[9] Restoring mobility to the restricted segment increases parasympathetic nerve fibers. A somatovisceral (muscle-organ) reflex is when a musculoskeletal ailment can lead to functional changes of an organ or immune function.

There is also some preliminary evidence of chiropractic aiding in gastrointestinal symptoms of autoimmune disease.[10] Mast cells or mucus-producing cells are directly stimulated by the sympathetic nerves. Mast cells play a role in the initiation of inflammation and also in the neuroimmune signaling that is responsible for the hypersensitization of airways and the gastrointestinal system.[11, 12, 13]

Research shows general improvements of symptoms associated with Crohn's[14] and IBS[15] from chiropractic manipulation. Some anecdotal stories include complete remission. This suggests that nerve flow to the digestive organs wasn't optimized.

Chiropractic also had benefits on subjective symptoms related to allergies and asthma,[16] and a case report showed chiropractic eliminated symptoms associated with Myasthenia Gravis.[17] Other systems in the body that are stimulated by an increase in sympathetic nervous system include: mast cells, mucus linings, bone marrow, sweat glands, arteries, endocrine system, immune organs, digestive system, cardiovascular system, pulmonary system, reproductive system, and the optic lens.

I want to be clear. I do not think chiropractic care can cure autoimmune disease. But in specific individuals where nerve flow to specific organs is significantly altered, it can play a larger role in their specific case of autoimmunity, which may have life-changing effects.

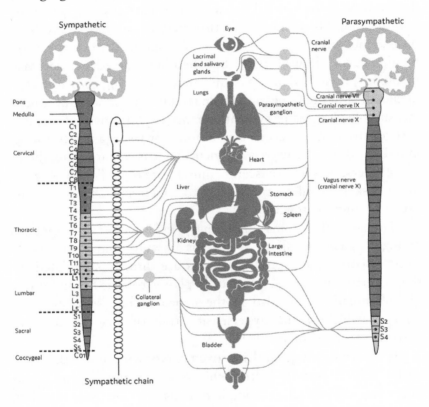

Chiropractic also has some interesting direct effects on the immune system, including that it has been shown to decrease the chance of ear infection in children.[18] Furthermore, it rapidly boosts white blood cell production and influences T and B lymphocytes, natural killer cells, antibodies, and phagocyte activity.[19, 20, 21] A study on HIV patients over a period of 6 months showed a 48 percent increase in CD4+ cells versus the other group which had an 8 percent decrease in CD4+ from baseline.[22] It seems as though reducing spinal restrictions is having a modulating effect on the immune system. Chiropractic manipulation also affects the release of hormones and peptides including oxytocin and neurotensin, both of which have analgesic effects, giving patients a feeling of well-being.[23]

Chiropractic treatment is extremely safe. There is no causal link between chiropractic cervical adjustments and strokes. A vertebral artery dissection (the stroke looked at with chiropractic treatment) occurs in 1 out of every 8.06 million office visits or 1 out of 48 chiropractic careers.[24] People with metabolic syndrome are most at risk for one of those events.

Acupuncture

Acupuncture is a part of Chinese medicine that has been around for thousands of years. It is the act of inserting very fine needles through the skin at specific points that are thought to have systematic effects by affecting the flow of Qi, or energy. In Western terms, you can think of this as stimulation of nerves, hormones, and blood flow. The belief is there are 12 meridians or channels around the body that are interconnected, 6 of which are yin energy, and 6 are yang energy. Whenever one becomes more dominant than the other, disease manifests. For example, needling an area on the hand that is on the same meridian as the kidney, could have effects on the kidney. Along the meridians exist hundreds of acupoints that are distinguished as areas of low electrical resistance and close proximity to nerve bundles. Acupuncture is used for both musculoskeletal issues and internal medicine.

There are different theories on what the meridians are based on. The one that resonates with me is that the Chinese meridians closely resemble the neuroembryological development of the body. After the egg is fertilized, the single cell begins to multiply and subtly specialize. The seemingly ambiguous and rapid proliferation of cells is actually highly organized. The cells begin to form chains that branch out with guidance from the cells' innate intelligence or DNA instructions coupled with environmental signaling.[25] In chiropractic care, referred pain is based on embryonic dermatomes. A trigger point in one muscle can lead to headaches or pain elsewhere.

Indifferent of the mechanism, what matters is that acupuncture works! For starters, it is effective for different types of pain, headaches, and stress, and therefore can be used to mitigate some of the symptoms of autoimmune disease. Acupuncture stimulates the release of opioids, endorphins, and serotonin, thus providing natural pain relief.[26] Blood flow is significantly increased in areas of blood stasis, which can help with symptoms associated with Rheumatoid Arthritis.[27] With regard to the influence on gut health, there is no robust research to back it up. Anecdotes are heavily reported to support techniques for constipation, diarrhea, IBS, or IBD.[28] Acupuncture also can have a calming effect by decreasing sympathetic nervous system overstimulation.[29] And, in itself, the act of penetrating the skin acts as a microtrauma, which stimulates the healing process local to the area. There is balance of yin and yang so some acupoints can actually have the opposite effect of what is desired.

In animal studies acupuncture was effective for treating Myasthenia Gravis.[30] Electro acupuncture is a form of acupuncture that sends an electric stimulus into the acupoint, causing a muscle fasciculation. Acupuncture is considered to be very safe. It can incorporate tools such as gua sha, cupping, or massage techniques, which will also release feel-good neurotransmitters, decrease pain, and increase range of motion.

Hypnotherapy

Hypnosis is a state of deep relaxation, concentration, and increased suggestibility. It is the bridge between the conscious and the subconscious mind. This state of mind can be used for therapeutic treatment. As explained in Chapter 5, each set of behaviors that you have is a memorized program in the brain. By getting a patient into a hypnotic state, the practitioner can help rewire some of the negative programs, habits, or beliefs. The obvious benefits are undoing triggering memories that may be stimulating chronic sympathetic overactivation or anxiety. For someone with a lot of traumas in their past, these experiences could be consistently playing a role in the stress contributing to their autoimmunity.

There is a lot of supportive evidence showing the effectiveness of hypnotherapy for IBD. Gut-focused hypnotherapy has been shown to decrease inflammation and increase quality of life in individuals with IBD, highlighting the gut-brain axis.[31, 32, 33, 34] Remember, the gut plays a role in most autoimmune diseases and may benefit from hypnotherapy. Gut-centered hypnotherapy includes patients being instructed to visualize and perform tactile techniques that normalize gastrointestinal function. The hypnosis allows access to control physiological functions that are not available during consciousness. It normalizes dysfunctional gut conditions and visceral signaling and increases parasympathetic stimulation of the Vagus nerve. You can visit a hypnotherapist or try listening to prerecorded tracks.

In summary, chiropractic care can be an effective tool for increasing nerve communication, which plays a role in immune signaling. Acupuncture can be used to decrease pain and stress. Hypnotherapy can rewire the brain and decrease dysfunction of the digestive organs. These therapies are not to be used without the foundation of the Kash Code, which includes diet and lifestyle changes.

NOTES

1   Porges, S. The polyvagal theory: new insights into adaptive reactions of the autonomic nervous system. Cleveland Clinical Journal of Medicine, April 2009; 2:S86–S90.

2   Alcedo, J. and Maier, W. (n.d.). *Sensory Influence on Homeostasis and Lifespan: Molecules and Circuits.* NCBI. Retrieved from https://www.ncbi .nlm.nih.gov/books/NBK25445.

3   Tomanek, R. J. and Lund, D. D. Degeneration of different types of skeletal muscle fibres. II. Immobilization. J Anat. 1974 Dec.;118(Pt 3):531–41.

4   Stokes, I.and Iatridis, J. Mechanical Conditions That Accelerate Intervertebral Disc Degeneration: Overload Versus Immobilization. Spine. 2004;29(23):2724–2732.

5   Ragab, A.; Escarcega, A.; Zdeblick, T. A quantitative analysis of strain at adjacent segments after segmental immobilization of the cervical spine. J Spinal Disord Tech. 2006;19(6):407–10.

6   Grassi, G.; Arenare, F.; Pieruzzi, F.; Brambilla, G.; Mancia, G. Sympathetic activation in cardiovascular and renal disease. J N Ephrol. 2009; 22: 190–195.

7   Manabe, N.; Tanaka, T.; Hata, J.; Kusunoki, H.; Haruma, K. Pathophysiology underlying irritable bowel syndrome from the viewpoint of dysfunction of autonomic nervous system acitivity. Journal of Smooth Muscle Research, 2009; 1: 15–23.

8   Person. (2007, March 13). *Special chiropractic adjustment lowers blood pressure among hypertensive patients with misaligned C1.* Special chiropractic adjustment lowers blood pressure among hypertensive patients with misaligned c1—UChicago Medicine. Retrieved from https://www .uchicagomedicine.org/forefront/news/special-chiropractic-adjustment -lowers-blood-pressure-among-hypertensive-patients-with-misaligned-c1.

9   Budgell, B., et al. Spinovisceral reflexes evoked by noxious and Innocuous stimulation of the lumbar spine. J Neuromusculoskel Syst; 1995;3:122–131.

10 Angus, K.; Asgharifar, S.; Gleberzon, B. (2015, June). *What effect does chiropractic treatment have on gastrointestinal (GI) disorders: A narrative review of the literature.* The Journal of the Canadian Chiropractic Association. Retrieved from https://www.ncbi.nlm.nih.gov/pmc/articles /PMC4486990.

11 Williams, R. M.; Bienenstock, J.; Stead, R. H. Mast cells: the neuroimmune connection. Chem Immunol. 1995;61:208–35.

12 McKay, D. M. and Bienenstock, J. The interaction between mast cells and nerves in the gastrointestinal tract. Immunol Today. 1994 Nov. 15 (11):533–8.

13 Bienenstock, J.; Tomioka, M.; Matsuda, H.; et al. The role of mast cells in inflammatory processes: evidence for nerve/mast cell interactions. Int Arch Allergy Appl Immunol. 1987;82 (3–4):238–43.

14 *Long term remission and alleviation of symptoms in allergy and crohn's disease patients following spinal adjustment for reduction of vertebral subluxations.* Vertebral Subluxation Research. (n.d.). Retrieved from https://www.vertebralsubluxationresearch.com/2017/09/10/long-term -remission-and-alleviation-of-symptoms-in-allergy-and-crohns-disease -patients-following-spinal-adjustment-for-reduction-of-vertebral -subluxations.

15 Angus, K.; Asgharifar, S.; Gleberzon, B. (2015, June). *What effect does chiropractic treatment have on gastrointestinal (GI) disorders: A narrative review of the literature.* The Journal of the Canadian Chiropractic Association. Retrieved from https://www.ncbi.nlm.nih.gov/pmc/articles /PMC4486990.

16 Kaminskyj, A.; Frazier, M.; Johnstone, K.; Gleberzon, B. J. (2010, March). *Chiropractic care for patients with asthma: A systematic review of the literature.* The Journal of the Canadian Chiropractic Association. Retrieved from https://www.ncbi.nlm.nih.gov/pmc/articles/PMC2829683.

17 Alcantara, J.; Plaugher, G.; and Araghi, H. J. (2003, Nov. 26). *Chiropractic care of a pediatric patient with myasthenia gravis.* Journal of Manipulative and Physiological Therapeutics. Retrieved from https://www.sciencedirect.com/science/article/pii/ S0161475403000721?casa_token=IkueFMpEE9kAAAAA%3AH wGbCmbb-E-m3j2_jQ4Fr3gsDezWfwXojd9GriBRMU4BQSm9 -Txu2ALYv5stTjATMpgTIJubBQ.

18 Van Breda, W. and Van Breda, J. A. (1989, Summer). "A Comparative Study of the Health Status of Children Raised Under the Health Care Models of Chiropractic and Allopathic Medicine." Chiropractic Research Journal, 101–103.

19 Chiropractic Journal of Australia. (1993). "The Effects of Chiropractic on the Immune System."

20 Brennan, P. and Hondras, M. (1989). "Priming of Neutrophils for Enhanced Respiratory Burst By Manipulation of the Thoracic Spine." International Conference on Spinal Manipulation, 160–163.

21 Pero, R. (1988). "Boosting Immunity Through Chiropractic." East-West Magazine.

22 Selano, J. L.; Hightower, B. C.; Pfleger, B.; Feeley-Collins, K.; Grostic, D. "The Effects of Specific Upper Cervical Adjustments on the CD4 Counts of HIV Positive Patients." The Chiro Research Journal; 3(1); 1994.

23 Plaza-Manzano, G.; Molina-Ortega, F.; Lomas-Vega, R.; Martínez-Amat, A.; Achalandabaso, A.; Hita-Contreras, F. (n.d.). *Changes in biochemical markers of pain perception and stress response after spinal manipulation.* The Journal of orthopaedic and sports physical therapy. Retrieved from https://pubmed.ncbi.nlm.nih.gov/24450367.

24 Carey, P.; Haldeman, S.; Townsend, M. (2001, Oct.). *Arterial dissections following cervical manipulation: the chiropractic experience.* NCBI. Retrieved from https://www.ncbi.nlm.nih.gov/pmc/articles/PMC81498.

25 Dorsher, P. T. and Chiang, P. (2018, April 1). *Neuroembryology of the Acupuncture Principal Meridians: Part 3. the head and Neck*. Medical acupuncture. Retrieved from https://www.ncbi.nlm.nih.gov/pmc/articles /PMC5908427.

26 Lee, M. S. and Ernst, E. (2011, Feb. 27). *Acupuncture for pain: An overview of Cochrane Reviews*. Chinese Journal of Integrative Medicine. Retrieved from https://link.springer.com/article/10.1007%2Fs11655-011-0665-7.

27 Z, S. (2001, Oct.). *A study of relation between rheumatoid arthritis (RA) and blood stasis--the effect of acupuncture promoting blood circulation to remove blood stasis]*. Europe PMC. Retrieved from https://europepmc.org /article/med/8706278.

28 Sung, J. J. Y. (2002, Nov. 1). *Acupuncture for gastrointestinal disorders: Myth or magic*. Gut. Retrieved from https://gut.bmj.com/content/51/5/617.1.full.

29 Li, Q.-Q.; Shi, G.-X.; Xu, Q.; Wang, J.; Liu, C.-Z.; Wang, L.-P. (2013). *Acupuncture effect and Central Autonomic Regulation*. Evidence-based complementary and alternative medicine : eCAM. Retrieved from https:// www.ncbi.nlm.nih.gov/pmc/articles/PMC3677642.

30 Pan, H. and Wang, H.-Feng. (2016, March). *"Warming yang and invigorating qi" acupuncture alters acetylcholine receptor expression in the neuromuscular junction of rats with experimental autoimmune myasthenia gravis*. NCBI. Retrieved from https://www.ncbi.nlm.nih.gov/pmc/articles /PMC4829013.

31 *Hypnotherapy for inflammatory bowel disease across the lifespan*. Taylor & Francis. (n.d.). Retrieved from https://www.tandfonline.com/doi /abs/10.1080/00029157.2015.1040112.

32 *The role of hypnotherapy for the treatment of inflammatory bowel diseases*. Taylor & Francis. (n.d.). Retrieved from https://www.tandfonline.com/doi /abs/10.1586/17474124.2014.917955.

33 *Treatment of inflammatory bowel disease: A role for hypnotherapy?* Taylor & Francis. (n.d.). Retrieved from https://www.tandfonline.com/doi /abs/10.1080/00207140802041884.

34 Abela, M. B. (2000, Sept. 14). *Hypnotherapy for crohn's disease: A promising complementary/alternative therapy*. Integrative Medicine. Retrieved from https://www.sciencedirect.com/science/article/abs/pii /S1096219000000056?via%3Dihub

CHAPTER 12

Supplements

S UPPLEMENTATION is a very important driver in helping you cross the finish line into autoimmune disease remission. Supplementation alone is not powerful enough to get the job done, but when done in concordance with the rest of the Kash Code, it will fit right into the keyhole and open the door toward health.

The supplements noted in this chapter are based on the premise that gut dysfunction is the biggest driver of autoimmune disease. Many of the supplements included here are intended to target gut health, while others target neutralizing free radicals in the body. I don't provide serving size or brand recommendations because supplements are case-by-case, and it's important to always start very small and work your way up. Starting at a dose too high can make your symptoms worse. Also keep in mind that, like food, supplements respond differently from one individual to another: they can make a positive difference in one person's autoimmune disease, but set someone else's back.

Digestion

Without proper enzymes, foods will not be broken down, leading to fermentation in the small intestines and contributing to dysbiosis. Enzyme levels can be tested for in a gut panel and may need to be introduced initially to better digest food and absorb nutrients for healing.

Enzymes to aid digestion

Hydrochloric acid	Protein digestion, stimulates mucous protection, and eliminates bacteria from food.
Pepsin	Digests protein and is often stacked with HCL.
Ox bile	Digests fats and helps eliminate gut infections.
Lipase	Digests fats.
Proteolytic enzymes	Important for breaking down proteins during a meal. Taken without food, the enzymes accelerate healing of skin, joints, and muscle.
Pancreatic enzymes	Digests fats, proteins, and carbohydrates.

Gut Barrier Integrity

Chapter 4 included information on the protocol for rebuilding a healthy gut through prebiotics, probiotics, and postbiotics. These can be used in conjunction with supplements that aid in increasing the mucosal barrier of the gut, soothing gut inflammation, and providing building blocks for the gut wall. Often, these ingredients are sold together in powders.

Aloe Vera	Herbal remedy that has immune modulating and gut-healing effects.[1]
Licorice root	Herbal remedy that soothes the gut lining.[2]
Slippery Elm	Herbal remedy that protects mucosal barrier function in gastrointestinal illness.[3]
L-glutamine	An amino acid that is a building block for restoring tight gap junctions in the intestinal wall.[4, 5, 6]
Colostrum or Serum Bovine Immunoglobulins	Colostrum is the first part of breast milk that is dense in growth factors and nutrients, including lactoferrin and IgG immunoglobulins. Colostrum and immunoglobulins reduce gut inflammation and provide growth factors to maintain tight gap junctions.[7, 8, 9]
N-acetylglucosamine (NAG)	Glycolated proteins provide a barrier from bacteria from the mucous layer to the intestinal lining. In gut issues these glycolated proteins are broken down. Supplementing with NAG serves as a building block that provides a binding site to beneficial bacteria on the lumen side of the mucous barrier.[10]
Marshmallow Root	An herbal remedy that soothes gut irritation and inflammation by stimulating mucous production.[11]

Quercetin	Quercetin is found in foods like onions, kale, and apples. It has antioxidants that have anti-inflammatory effects and stabilize mast cells; it also has counteracted glutathione deficiencies in colonic inflammation in animal studies. Mast cells in the colon play a role in causing leaky gut, and Quercetin has sealing effects on the gut-gap juctions.[12, 13]
Mastic Gum	Mastic is a gum that comes from trees on the Greek island of Chios. It can be chewed or consumed in pill form. Mastic gum has some antibiotic benefits in the mouth and anti-inflammatory and soothing effects in the gut.[14] The gum comes in very small balls. I enjoy chewing it after meals.

Natural Anti-Inflammatories

Controlling inflammation is key for allowing your body to digest food and jumpstart the healing process. These supplements are not necessarily to be used in the long term since, just like pharmaceutical agents, long-term use of herbal supplements can have side effects and lose effectiveness. They should be used in the beginning phases of healing and during flares.

CBD[15, 16]
Liposomal Turmeric[17]
Ginger[18]
Sustained release peppermint oil[19]

Micronutrients

Zinc	Zinc deficiencies cause all sorts of immune dysregulation. Supplementation with zinc has been shown to help seal up the intestinal walls.[20, 21]
Vitamin D3	Low serum Vitamin D can contribute to multiple autoimmune diseases. If supplemented with vitamin D3, it should be stacked with vitamin K2 to prevent arterial calcification.[22]
Desiccated Organs	Glandular theory is based on consuming the organ that is injured in your own body to provide building blocks or nutrients needed to heal it. Primitive tribes have used this wisdom around the world. Organs are the most nutrient-dense foods found in nature and provide many micronutrients and peptides that are of great value to the body. Using this principal for systematic immunity, you can supplement with spleen and thymus. In my case, I supplemented with desiccated intestines. In the case of thyroid diseases, one can supplement with thyroid. There is not much to back up these claims besides an old radioisotope study.[23]

Peptides / Hormones

Hormones are amino acids linked together in a sophisticated chain. Many of the complex proteins we digest are broken down and restricted to form different chains. These chains become part of the language of cells.

Smaller portions of a hormone can be classified as peptides. Peptides are generally more specific in action with fewer side effects. These peptide chains are chemical instructions for cells to perform a specific action such as healing. These are the type of peptides used for therapeutic effects. Peptides can be purchased directly or through doctors that have relationships with compounding pharmacies. Peptides can be delivered through injection, patches, topicals, orally, or as suppositories.

Many peptides are considered safe, but experimental. They often do not get the research funding that is deserved because of difficulties in patentability. Although these peptides are made and produced in our bodies, there are no long-term studies to show the safety of injecting synthetic isolated amounts of them into tissues. Peptides are going to be at the forefront of healing therapies in the future. Following is a list of the most commonly used and well-known therapeutic peptides.

Types of peptides

BPC-157	Body protective compound 157 is a peptide that gives instructions for cellular healing, especially in the gut. Animal studies have shown BPC-157 to protect and heal inflamed intestinal lining.[24] BPC-157 is also effective for speeding up joint and tendon healing.[25]
TB-500	Thymosin-Beta 4 is a peptide made from the thymus gland. Many individuals with autoimmune disease have a dysfunctional or underperforming thymus, so there may be a deficiency in production of this peptide. TB-500 has been shown to speed up the healing process,[26] regenerate organs,[27] and regenerate blood vessels.[28]
GPK-CU	Copper zinc peptide stimulates blood vessels and nerve growth, and increases collagen and elastin production. It can improve repair of the stomach lining and other organs.[29] This may be the best peptide for skin conditions.

LL-37	Antimicrobial peptide LL-37 is used as a mechanism against bacterial and fungal invasion. It can be used to help treat dysbiosis and break down the biofilms that house microbes in the gut.[30] Before feeling better, you may experience an initial worsening of symptoms from a die-off in bacteria.
Secretin/ Oxytocin	Secretin is a hormone that stimulates secretions of the liver and pancreas. Oxytocin is known as the love hormone and is released to stimulate lactation and affectionate behavior. Oxytocin also delays gastric emptying and slows intestinal transit. The combination of the two hormones has been shown to decrease intestinal inflammation.[31, 32]
Melatonin	The circadian rhythm hormone plays a role in modulating the immune system and can aid in decreasing the severity of autoimmune symptoms.[33]
Larazotide	Larazotide is a peptide that tightens gap junctions in the gut and decreases inflammatory response of gluten in Celiac disease.[34]

Neutralize Free Radicals

As a quick refresher, free radicals are unstable molecules formed by stress and can cause further damaging cascades, especially when they reach high levels as seen in autoimmune disease. Neutralizing free radicals prevents further DNA damage and inflammation.

Some choices to neutralize free radicals

Nicotinamide Adenine Dinucleotide (NAD)	NAD is a coenzyme in energy production. NAD levels decrease as we age and are depleted in chronic diseases.[35] NAD can be administered through IV, nasal sprays, transdermal patches, or oral precursors.
Glutathione	Glutathione promotes T-regulatory cell production and differentiation. Glutathione levels have been shown to be low in patients with autoimmune disease.[36] Glutathione can be administered through injection, transdermal patches, or in liposomal forms.
Hydrogen-Enriched Water	Hydrogen-enriched water increases free radical scavenging and has anti-inflammatory effects. Special water filters can infuse hydrogen into the water. Also, hydrogen tablets can be dissolved in drinking water or bathwater. Hydrogen-infused water has the best effect when used in pulses rather than drinking it consistently throughout the day.[37] Avoid drinking hydrogen-enriched water before, during, or after meals because of its alkalizing effect on the stomach.

By no means should you be taking all of these supplements at the same time. They have been explained so that they can be experimented with during different phases of healing to see if they can help with signs and symptoms of your disease. Dosing, frequency, and timing as well as the type of supplement should be catered to the individual.

NOTES

1   *Randomized, double-blind, placebo-controlled trial of oral aloe vera gel for active ulcerative colitis.* (n.d.). Retrieved from https://onlinelibrary .wiley.com/doi/epdf/10.1111/j.1365-2036.2004.01902.x.

2   Peterson, C. T.; Sharma, V.; Uchitel, S.; Denniston, K.; Chopra, D.; Mills, P. J.; Peterson, S. N. (2018, July). *Prebiotic potential of herbal medicines used in digestive health and disease.* Journal of alternative and complementary medicine (New York, N.Y.). Retrieved from https://www.ncbi.nlm.nih.gov /pmc/articles/PMC6065514.

3   Peterson, C. T.; Sharma, V.; Uchitel, S.; Denniston, K.; Chopra, D.; Mills, P. J.; Peterson, S. N. (2018, July). *Prebiotic potential of herbal medicines used in digestive health and disease.* Journal of alternative and complementary medicine (New York, N.Y.). Retrieved from https://www.ncbi.nlm.nih.gov /pmc/articles/PMC6065514.

4   Bertrand, J.; Ghouzali, I.; Guérin, C.; Bôle-Feysot, C.; Gouteux, M.; Déchelotte, P.; Ducrotté, P.; Coëffier, M. (2016, Nov.). *Glutamine restores tight junction protein claudin-1 expression in colonic mucosa of patients with diarrhea-predominant irritable bowel syndrome.* JPEN. Journal of parenteral and enteral nutrition. Retrieved from https://www.ncbi.nlm.nih .gov/pubmed/25972430.

5   Benjamin, J.; Makharia, G.; Ahuja, V.; Anand Rajan, K. D.; Kalaivani, M.; Gupta, S. D.; Joshi, Y. K. (2012, April). *Glutamine and whey protein improve intestinal permeability and morphology in patients with crohn's disease: A randomized controlled trial.* Digestive diseases and sciences. Retrieved from https://www.ncbi.nlm.nih.gov/pubmed/22038507.

6   Den Hond, E.; Hiele, M.; Peeters, M.; Ghoos, Y.; Rutgeerts, P. (1999). *Effect of long-term oral glutamine supplements on small intestinal permeability in patients with Crohn's disease.* JPEN. https://www.ncbi.nlm.nih.gov /pubmed/9888411.

7   Otsuki, K.; Yoda, A.; Saito, H.; Mitsuhashi, Y.; Toma, Y.; Shimizu, Y.; Yanaihara, T. (n.d.). *Amniotic fluid lactoferrin in intrauterine infection.* Placenta. Retrieved from https://pubmed.ncbi.nlm.nih.gov/10195738.

8   Blais, A.; Fan, C.; Voisin, T.; Aattouri, N.; Dubarry, M.; Blachier, F.; Tomé, D. (n.d.). *Effects of lactoferrin on intestinal epithelial cell growth and differentiation: An in vivo and in vitro study.* Biometals : an international journal on the role of metal ions in biology, biochemistry, and medicine. Retrieved from https://pubmed.ncbi.nlm.nih.gov/25082351.

9   Shafran, I.; Burgunder, P.; Wei, D.; Young, H. E.; Klein, G.; Burnett, B. P.
     (2015, Nov.). *Management of inflammatory bowel disease with oral serum-
     derived bovine immunoglobulin.* Therapeutic advances in gastroenterology.
     Retrieved from https://www.ncbi.nlm.nih.gov/pmc/articles/PMC4622288.

10   Zhu, A. Z. X.; Zhu, A; the A. A. Z. X.; Zhu, A. Z. X.; Patel, I.; Hidalgo,
     M.; Gandhi, V. (n.d.). *N-acetylglucosamine for treatment of inflammatory
     bowel disease.* Natural Medicine Journal. Retrieved from https://www
     .naturalmedicinejournal.com/journal/2015-04/n-acetylglucosamine
     -treatment-inflammatory-bowel-disease.

11   Deters, A.; Zippel, J.; Hellenbrand, N.; Pappai, D.; Possemeyer, C.;
     Hensel, A. (2009, Sept. 30). *Aqueous extracts and polysaccharides from
     marshmallow roots (Althea officinalis L.): Cellular internalisation and
     stimulation of cell physiology of human epithelial cells in vitro.* Journal
     of Ethnopharmacology. Retrieved from https://www.sciencedirect.com
     /science/article/abs/pii/S0378874109006102.

12   J;, P. F. L. B. A. D. B. (n.d.). *Mucosal mast cells. III. effect of quercetin and
     other flavonoids on antigen-induced histamine secretion from rat intestinal
     mast cells.* The Journal of allergy and clinical immunology. Retrieved from
     https://pubmed.ncbi.nlm.nih.gov/6202731.

13   Suzuki, T. and Hara, H. (2010, Dec. 16). *Role of flavonoids in intestinal
     tight junction regulation.* The Journal of Nutritional Biochemistry.
     Retrieved   from   https://www.sciencedirect.com/science/article/pii
     /S0955286310001877.

14   Triantafyllidi, A.; Xanthos, T.; Papalois, A.; Triantafillidis, J. K. (2015).
     Herbal and plant therapy in patients with inflammatory bowel disease.
     Annals of gastroenterology. Retrieved from https://www.ncbi.nlm.nih.gov
     /pmc/articles/PMC4367210.

15   Pauli, C. S.; Conroy, M.; Vanden Heuvel, B. D.; Park, S.-H. (2020, Feb. 25).
     Cannabidiol drugs clinical trial outcomes and adverse effects. Frontiers in
     pharmacology. Retrieved from https://www.ncbi.nlm.nih.gov/pmc/articles
     /PMC7053164.

16   Atalay, S.; Jarocka-Karpowicz, I.; Skrzydlewska, E. (2019, Dec. 25).
     Antioxidative   and   anti-inflammatory   properties   of   Cannabidiol.
     Antioxidants (Basel, Switzerland). Retrieved from https://www.ncbi.nlm
     .nih.gov/pmc/articles/PMC7023045.

17   Toden, S. and Goel, A. (2017, Dec.). *The holy grail of curcumin and its
     efficacy in various diseases: Is bioavailability truly a big concern?* Journal
     of restorative medicine. Retrieved from https://www.ncbi.nlm.nih.gov
     /pmc/articles/PMC6424351.

18   Mashhadi, N. S.; Ghiasvand, R.; Askari, G.; Hariri, M.; Darvishi, L.; Mofid,
     M. R. (2013, April). *Anti-oxidative and anti-inflammatory effects of ginger
     in health and physical activity: Review of current evidence.* International
     journal of preventive medicine. Retrieved from https://www.ncbi.nlm.nih
     .gov/pmc/articles/PMC3665023.

19   Alammar, N.; Wang, L.; Saberi, B.; Nanavati, J.; Holtmann, G.; Shinohara,
     R. T.; Mullin, G. E. (2019, Jan. 17). *The impact of peppermint oil on*

The irritable bowel syndrome: A meta-analysis of the pooled clinical data. BMC complementary and alternative medicine. Retrieved from https://www.ncbi.nlm.nih.gov/pmc/articles/PMC6337770.

20 Sturniolo, G. C.; Di Leo, V.; Ferronato, A.; D'Odorico, A.; D'Incà, R. (2001, May). *Zinc supplementation tightens "leaky gut" in crohn's disease.* Inflammatory bowel diseases. Retrieved from https://www.ncbi.nlm.nih.gov/pubmed/11383597.

21 Sturniolo, G. C.; Fries, W.; Mazzon, E.; Di Leo, V.; Barollo, M.; D'inca, R. (2002, May). *Effect of zinc supplementation on intestinal permeability in experimental colitis.* The Journal of laboratory and clinical medicine. Retrieved from https://www.ncbi.nlm.nih.gov/pubmed/12032492.

22 Yang, C.-Y.; Leung, P. S. C.; Adamopoulos, I. E.; Gershwin, M. E. (2013, Oct.). *The implication of Vitamin D and autoimmunity: A comprehensive review.* Clinical reviews in allergy & immunology. Retrieved from https://www.ncbi.nlm.nih.gov/pmc/articles/PMC6047889.

23 Hemmings, W. W. and Williams, E. W. (1978). Transport of large breakdown products of dietary protein through the gut wall. *Gut,* 715–723.

24 Sikiric. P.; Seiwerth, S.; Rucman, R.; Turkovic, B.; Rokotov, D. S.; Brcic, L.; Sever, M.; Klicek, R.; Radic, B.; Drmic, D.; Ilic, S.; Kolenc, D.; Stambolija, V.; Zoricic, Z.; Vrcic, H.; Sebecic, B. (n.d.). *Focus on ulcerative colitis: Stable gastric pentadecapeptide BPC 157.* Current medicinal chemistry. Retrieved from https://pubmed.ncbi.nlm.nih.gov/22300085.

25 Chang, C. H.; Tsai, W. C.; Lin, M. S.; Hsu, Y. H.; Pang, J. H. (n.d.). *The promoting effect of pentadecapeptide BPC 157 on tendon healing involves tendon outgrowth, cell survival, and cell migration.* Journal of applied physiology (Bethesda, Md. : 1985). Retrieved from https://pubmed.ncbi.nlm.nih.gov/21030672.

26 Sosne, G.; Qiu, P.; Kurpakus-Wheater, M. (2007, Sept.). *Thymosin beta 4: A novel corneal wound healing and anti-inflammatory agent.* Clinical ophthalmology (Auckland, N.Z.). Retrieved from https://www.ncbi.nlm.nih.gov/pmc/articles/PMC2701135.

27 Aurora, A. B. and Olson, E. N. (2014, July 3). *Immune modulation of stem cells and regeneration.* Cell stem cell. Retrieved from https://www.ncbi.nlm.nih.gov/pmc/articles/PMC4131296.

28 Wei, C.; Kim, I. K.; Li, L.; Wu, L.; Gupta, S. (n.d.). *Thymosin beta 4 protects mice from monocrotaline-induced pulmonary hypertension and right ventricular hypertrophy.* PloS one. Retrieved from https://pubmed.ncbi.nlm.nih.gov/25412097.

29 Pickart, L. and Margolina, A. (2018, July 7). *Regenerative and protective actions of the GHK-cu peptide in the light of the new Gene Data.* International journal of molecular sciences. Retrieved from https://www.ncbi.nlm.nih.gov/pmc/articles/PMC6073405.

30 Duplantier, A. J. and van Hoek, M. L. (1AD, Jan. 1). *The human cathelicidin antimicrobial peptide LL-37 as a potential treatment for polymicrobial*

infected wounds. Frontiers. Retrieved from https://www.frontiersin.org /articles/10.3389/fimmu.2013.00143/full.

31 Welch, M. G.; Anwar, M.; Chang, C. Y.; Gross, K. J.; Ruggiero, D. A.; Tamir, H.; Gershon, M. D. (2010, June). *Combined administration of secretin and oxytocin inhibits chronic colitis and associated activation of forebrain neurons.* Neurogastroenterology and motility : the official journal of the European Gastrointestinal Motility Society. Retrieved from https://www.ncbi.nlm.nih.gov/pmc/articles/PMC3068601.

32 Tang, Y.; Shi, Y.; Gao, Y.; Xu, X.; Han, T.; Li, J.; Liu, C. (2019, Sept. 19). *Oxytocin system alleviates intestinal inflammation by regulating macrophages polarization in experimental colitis.* Portland Press. Retrieved from https://portlandpress.com/clinsci/article-abstract /133/18/1977/220436/Oxytocin-system-alleviates-intestinal -inflammation?redirectedFrom=fulltext.

33 Lin, G.-J.; Huang, S.-H.; Chen, S.-J.; Wang, C.-H.; Chang, D.-M.; Sytwu, H.-K. (2013, May 31). *Modulation by melatonin of the pathogenesis of inflammatory autoimmune diseases.* International journal of molecular sciences. Retrieved from https://www.ncbi.nlm.nih.gov/pmc/articles /PMC3709754.

34 Stein, J. and Schuppan, D. (2014, June). *Coeliac disease - new pathophysiological findings and their implications for therapy.* Viszeralmedizin. Retrieved from https://www.ncbi.nlm.nih.gov/pmc /articles/PMC4513807.

35 *The role of NAD+ in the pathogenesis of rheumatoid arthritis.* European Medical Journal. (2021, July 16). Retrieved from https://www.emjreviews .com/rheumatology/article/the-role-of-nicotinamide-adenine-dinucleotide -in-the-pathogenesis-of-rheumatoid-arthritis-potential-implications-for -treatment.

36 R;, P. C. D. C. C. P. (n.d.). *Glutathione: A key player in autoimmunity.* Autoimmunity reviews. Retrieved from https://pubmed.ncbi.nlm.nih .gov/19393193.

37 *Hydrogen: An Emerging Medical Gas.* Molecular Hydrogen Institute. (n.d.). Retrieved from http://www.molecularhydrogeninstitute.com /hydrogen-an-emerging-medical-gas.

CHAPTER 13

The Kash Code
User Manual

THE KASH CODE was designed as a tool for individuals suffering from autoimmune disease to learn about radical diet and lifestyle changes that can have a life-changing effect on their condition. It is a resource compiled of all of my research organized in such a way that individuals can be made aware of its existence, educated on it, and then, if interested, they can explore more about a therapy or supplement and discuss it with their doctor. It is meant to provide a personalized approach to treating the root cause of your disease, in a way that conventional medicine does not.

What may reverse one individual's autoimmune disease may not be enough of a lifestyle change to reverse someone else's. The Kash Code offers a calculated and science-based trial-and-error approach. One person can simply remove gluten while someone else can go on the strictest elimination diet and still have to continue experimenting. Furthermore, it is important to take small steps. If you try everything all at once, it may be unsustainable for the long term. Your own method can be customized through different references you have read throughout the book. You can attempt the suggestions on your own, but I recommend working with a functional medicine professional who can guide you and order/interpret labs. The method can be used concomitantly with drugs/pharmaceuticals prescribed by your doctor with the goal of eventually reducing the dose or no longer needing them.

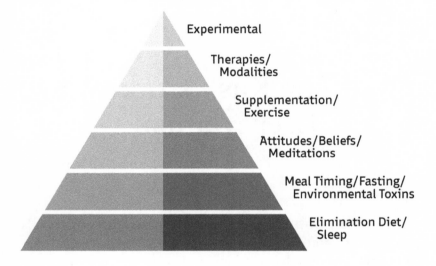

This pyramid provides an order of operations that I deem most important to resolving autoimmune disease. The premise is based on my theory that compounding stress to the system and the absence of proper immune signaling is the recipe for autoimmune disease. The very foundation of the pyramid includes elimination diet and sleep. The biggest lever to healing is finding out what foods contribute to an inflammatory immune response and providing yourself with adequate sleep for restoration and recovery.

What we put into our bodies is the highest accumulation of stress that we receive. This occurs where the majority of our immune system cells reside. By eliminating foods that are potentially triggering, our stomach lining has an opportunity to heal, our gut microbe populations can fall back into homeostasis, and our nutrient absorption increases. The gut microbes produce chemical signals that communicate with all the other organs of the body. Dysbiosis, the presence of an unideal gut microbiome, contributes to a cycle of inflammation that both damages the gut lining and provides systematic inflammatory signals. If we continue to insult our insides, the power of the rest of the pyramid will be inhibited.

For example, let's say you have removed trigger foods, but you are not receiving ample amount of sleep or your circadian rhythm is out of sync; this is going to throw a wrench into proper hormonal and immune system signaling, as it prevents the release of healing peptides and hormones, while jacking up stress hormones. Lack of sleep disrupts the relationship between your gut bacteria and your body. The absence of adequate quality sleep will make it impossible for the body to facilitate healing and achieve optimal immune signaling. The combination of the elimination diet and quality sleep rhythms should be something you are unwilling to compromise on in your pursuit back to health.

The next layer of the pyramid is fasting/meal timing/environmental toxins.

Various forms of fasting that are right for you will provide time for your digestive system to relax and boost the hormones needed for healing. Cyclical prolonged fasting will allow for the digestion and recycling of hyperactive white blood cells responsible for autoimmune disease and a robust increase in stem cells in order to manufacture new healthy cells. The timing of meals is also very important; ceasing feeding 4 hours before bed will increase deep sleep, detoxification, autophagy, and glymphatic drainage.

Environmental toxins can also be a large contributor toward your autoimmune disease. Eliminating plastics, heavy metals, and pesticides from food, water, and cosmetic/hygienic products will free up space in the body's stress bank. Radiation and EMFs can also be a concern and warrant action to minimize exposure.

The third layer of the pyramid includes attitudes, beliefs, and meditation. Humans are exposed to 24 hours nonstop stress in today's world when, in nature, stress might have existed in brief bouts of fight or flight. Constantly being in a stressed state is going to wobble the body out of immune homeostasis. It is important that we find ways to de-stress, even if it is in small snacks throughout the day. It is also critical that one believes that they have the power to control what happens in their life. They have control of their choices, and that can shape their future. Hopelessness has no room in healing from autoimmune disease. Every thought produces real-time chemical signals that affect all the cells in your body. A positive outlook and attitude as well as loving yourself are prerequisites for winning back your body. Individuals with PTSD or other psychological/mental illness may lower this layer closer to the base of the pyramid as it may be contributing more to their disease than for others.

The fourth layer is supplementation. This layer is highly individualized. The first step may include supplementing with any nutrients that may be deficient in the body (vitamin D, zinc, folate, etc.), digestive enzymes and HCL, building blocks for the gut, and anti-inflammatories. Next, prebiotics, probiotics, postbiotics, and herbs can be carefully selected and tested. Finally, supplements that can help accelerate healing and neutralize free radicals can be used, including peptides, NAD, or glutathione.

Exercise is also placed at this layer; however, its importance should precede many of the supplements. Acute exercise is an environmental stressor that signals your body to become more resilient and produces endogenous antioxidants, builds up cartilage, bone, and nerves, and produces feel-good neurotransmitters. Different modes of exercise can be performed for different ranges of autoimmune disease.

The fifth layer of the pyramid includes professional therapies and healing modalities. Chiropractic can be a powerful tool for individuals who have severe restrictions especially in the spine, by freeing nerve flow to effective organs while also decreasing pain associated with autoimmune disease. Acupuncture is a professional therapy that's been around for thousands of years for combating pain, decreasing overactivated sympathetic drive, and stimulating a healing effect.

The first healing modalities to include are sauna, red light, cryotherapy, breath work, UV, and grounding. The more sophisticated modality that can be introduced when your body still needs something more powerful to push the needle is HBOT. All of these tools have different mechanisms and are condition-dependent.

The very top of the pyramid is for experimental therapies. These may be needed when you are still not receiving enough relief to live a high-quality life and are willing to experiment where there is not enough current research and may be very expensive. Some therapies that I would include as experimental include FMT, blood irradiation, Helminthic therapy, ozone, stem cells, and anything else out there that has preliminary or mixed evidence with an added layer of risk.

These layers of the Kash Code can be mixed and matched to suit the individual. As a whole, most humans are limited to speaking one language. However, the cells of your body speak thousands. They can communicate with other bacteria, EMFs, hormones, pressure, chemicals, and more. Understanding and utilizing these mechanisms you can turn off the genes for disease and turn on the genes for robust health.

Good luck with the journey and remember there is no purpose to life in the absence of obstacles to overcome!

Index

About the Author

*D*r. Colby Kash graduated *cum laude* from the University of Florida's College of Health and Human Performance with a Bachelor's in Applied Physiology and Kinesiology. He then went on to achieve his Doctor of Chiropractic at the Northeast College of Health Sciences as class president. Concurrently, he earned a Master of Science in Applied Clinical Nutrition. He continued to follow his passion within health, wellness, and longevity by pursuing the ADAPT Functional Medicine certification, the American College of Sports Medicine Exercise Physiologist Certification, the National Academy of Sports Medicine Personal Training Certification, as well as additional continuing education on health-related topics.

Dr. Kash pivoted out of clinical practice in order to scale his skillset and passion for healthcare by cofounding biotechnology companies dedicated to bringing novel technologies to life that increase the human health span. Dr. Kash lectures on healthcare related topics.

CPSIA information can be obtained
at www.ICGtesting.com
Printed in the USA
BVHW082317211222
654816BV00004B/78